Let Food Be Thy Medicine

Resources

The Kushi Institute — A center for macrobiotic and holistic studies located in the Berkshire mountains of western Massachusetts with affiliates in Amsterdam and Milan and extension programs in various North American cities. In "A New Medicine for Humanity," Michio Kushi offers ongoing seminars on the origin and development of health, the relation of diet and degenerative disease, and the reorientation of society in a healthier, more peaceful direction. For information, contact the Kushi Institute, Box 7, Becket, MA 01223 (413) 623-5741.

One Peaceful World — One Peaceful World is an international information network and friendship society of individuals, families, educational centers, organic farmers, teachers, parents and children, authors and artists, homemakers and business people, and others devoted to the realization of one healthy, peaceful world. Activities include educational and spiritual tours, assemblies and forums, international food aid and development, and publishing. For membership information, contact: One Peaceful World, Box 10, Becket MA 01223 (413) 623-2322.

Alex Jack is a journalist, author, and teacher. He has served as editor-in-chief of the *East West Journal*, director of the Kushi Institute of the Berkshires, and coordinator of One Peaceful World. He has taught at the New England Acupuncture Center, the Natural Organic Farmers Association, and the Cardiology Center of St. Petersburg. With Michio Kushi, he is the co-author of *The Cancer-Prevention Diet, Diet for a Strong Heart*, and *One Peaceful World*. He lives with his wife and daughter in western Massachusetts.

Let Food Be Thy Medicine

185 Scientific Studies Showing the
Physical, Mental, and Environmental
Benefits of Whole Foods

Edited by Alex Jack

One Peaceful World Press
Becket, Massachusetts

For Jon, Michael, Molly, Masha, and the next generation.

Published by One Peaceful World, Becket, MA

For further information on mail-order sales, wholesale or retail dis-
counts, distribution, translations, and foreign rights, please contact
the publisher:

One Peaceful World Press
P.O. Box 10
308 Leland Road
Becket, MA 01223
U.S.A.

Telephone (413) 623-2322
Fax (413) 623-8827

First edition: September 1991
10 9 8 7 6 5 4 3 2

Printed in U.S.A.

Contents

Tables & Charts

Introduction

"Let food be thy medicine and thy medicine food."
— Hippocrates

For thousands of years, the human family has been living free from degenerative disease in harmony with nature. Today, about 90 percent of people in modern society die from heart disease, cancer, diabetes, Alzheimer's disease, AIDS, and other chronic illnesses. These diseases are primarily the result of our imbalanced modern way of life, especially the modern way of eating which is high in fat and sugar, low in fiber, and laden with chemicals.

Nearly 2500 years ago in ancient Greece, Hippocrates, the Father of Medicine, taught that proper food was the foundation of human health and happiness. This is enshrined in the original Hippocratic Oath:

I will apply dietetic measures for the benefit of the sick according to my ability and judgment; I will keep them from harm and injustice.

Hippocrates recommended a way of eating based principally on barley, wheat, and other whole cereal grains that grew in the Hellenistic world. Traditional physicians in the Far East, the Middle East, India, Africa, the Americas, and other cultures also passed along dietary wisdom based on the grains, vegetables, and other predominantly plant-quality foods native to their environment. For many generations, the relation between food and disease has been neglected in modern society. In medical schools, the Hippocratic Oath was rewritten. The word "dietetic" was taken out — we might say, surgically removed! Upon graduation, medical students today pledge to apply unspecified "measures for the benefit of the sick."

Now after several centuries in which drugs and surgery have dominated medical treatment, modern science and medicine are rediscovering the power of food to maintain optimal health and happiness and to prevent and relieve illness. They are also beginning to recognize that the way we eat has a profound impact on mental and psychological health, as well as on the health of society and the environment.

This book summarizes the major scientific studies, medical guidelines, nutritional findings, and agricultural and ecological reports associating whole, natural foods with personal and planetary health. A few studies also have been included noting the harmful effects of white flour, white rice, dairy food, meat, and other animal products for which healthy alternative sources of complex carbohydrates, vegetable protein, calcium, iron, or other nutrients are readily available.

Many of these studies focus on the way of eating in the remaining traditional societies around the world where modern sicknesses are rare or unknown. Others involve vegetarians, vegans, and others avoiding or eliminating animal food from their diet. The majority have been inspired by the international macrobiotic community, under the leadership of Michio and Aveline Kushi. For the last thirty years, the Kushis and their associates have worked to reverse modern society's trend toward biological degeneration and spearheaded the educational movement to inform the public about the relation of diet and degenerative disease. (See the Appendix for a summary of macrobiotic dietary recommendations.)

In the late 1970s and early 1980s, government commissions, health ministries, and national and international medical associations began issuing dietary guidelines for the first time calling for substantial reductions in daily consumption of saturated fat and dietary cholesterol, sugar and other refined carbohydrates, and highly processed foods, as well as corresponding increases in whole grains and their products, fresh vegetables and fruit, and other natural foods. Every year the recommended volume of saturated fat, animal protein, and sugar has gradually decreased and the amount of fiber, complex carbohydrates, and vegetable-quality protein has gradually risen.

Modern medicine is clearly moving in a healthier direction.

This spring, the U.S. Department of Agriculture announced that the Four Basic Food Groups, the heart of the modern nutritional canon for the last two generations, would undergo major surgery. The Food Wheel that schoolchildren have grown up with since the 1950s would be replaced with an Eating Right Pyramid that puts whole grains (including bread, rice, cereal, and pasta) on the broad foundation, vegetables and fruits on the next level, high protein products (including meat, dairy, fish, beans, and nuts) in a small section near the top, and fats, oils, and sweets at the peak with a warning to use sparingly. After last-minute opposition by the beef and dairy industries, the U.S.D.A. postponed plans to distribute a million posters of the Pyramid to schools. While it may take another few years for modern society to implement even moderate dietary guidelines, essentially the diet and health revolution is over.

During the 1990s and early 21st century, we can expect these trends:

• Heart attacks, strokes, and other cardiovascular diseases will continue to drop sharply.

• Cancer rates in the U.S. and other industrial societies will begin to decline for the first time, especially those of the lung, colon, and breast, as fat consumption drops and fiber intake rises.

• Diet and nutrition will emerge as the key factors in the development of AIDS and other immune-deficiency diseases.

• Populations exposed to nuclear radiation, pollution, and other environmental toxins will incorporate miso soup, sea vegetables, and other foods that are protective against contaminants into their daily diets.

• Healthier foods will be introduced into schools, hospitals, clinics, prisons, businesses, and other institutions, leading to less aggressive and antisocial behavior, increased efficiency and cooperation, and better human relations.

• Organic and natural agriculture will gradually replace chemical agriculture and become recognized as inseparable from preserving the environment and maintaining planetary health.

As T. Colin Campbell and Chen Junshi, the directors of the China Health Study, observed, "The occurrence of most human diseases is usually the result of exposure to many factors occurring over a long period of time." Modern medicine's analytic approach — isolating one nutrient or component and seeking a specific cause-and-effect mechanism — must be balanced by the synthetic approach in which the balance of the diet as a whole, as well as its relation to lifestyle and environmental factors, is considered. In the future, dietary and nutritional research methods will also need to pay more attention to food quality. For example, are the foods whole or refined? Traditionally processed or artificially processed? Organically or chemically grown? Consumed seasonally or year round? Beside scientific and medical studies, there are other avenues to knowledge and understanding, including cultural tradition, spiritual development, literary and artistic creation, and intuition and self-reflection. The medicine of the future will integrate ancient and modern, Eastern and Western, synthetic and analytic, and other complementary strands that make up the tapestry of our daily lives. As Campbell and Junshi remind us, we need always to keep in mind "the big picture" — or what has traditionally been called the macrobiotic view.*

The editor would like to thank Michio and Aveline Kushi for their inspiration and leadership in helping to create a new medicine for humanity; the many diet and health researchers whose hard work and findings are summarized in this volume including William Castelli, Martha Cottrell, Lawrence Kushi, Tom Monte, Mark Mead, and Vivien Newbold; the modern medical profession which is issuing more commonsense dietary guidelines with each passing year (and it is hoped soon will put dietary guidance back into the Hippocratic Oath); the many laboratory animals that gave their lives to help us remember our true origin in the vegetal kingdom; my associates here in Becket, especially Edward and Wendy Esko, Charles and Marlene Millman, Michael and Alice Joutras, and Lynda Shoup, for their support and encouragement; and my wife, Gale, whose love and wonderful daily cooking helps keep me focused on our common dream of a healthy, peaceful world.

Alex Jack
Becket, Massachusetts
May 25, 1991

---

* Interestingly, the term *makrobios* — macrobiotic — was first used by Hippocrates in his essay *Air, Water, Places*. From ancient Greece, the term gradually spread around the world as a synonym for longevity and a healthy, peaceful life.

1

Traditional Wisdom

Traditional wisdom has been passed down the generations in myth, legend, symbol, and stone. In written form, traditional science and medicine date back to the Hippocratic teachings in the West and the Yellow Emperor's Classic in the Far East. In modern times, the commonsense dietary practices of our ancestors, great-grandparents, and grandparents has been shown in the work of Renaissance and Enlightenment health reformers, in the study of traditional societies by early 20th century medical and scientific pioneers, and in present-day research on the way of eating in paleolithic times and among primitive cultures today. The emerging consensus is that a balanced diet, based on whole cereal grains, beans and legumes, fresh vegetables from land and sea, and a small condiment-sized use of animal food has maintained the usual good health of the human family for endless generations.

1. Hippocrates

Nearly twenty-five hundred years ago, Hippocrates, the Father of Medicine, taught a natural healing method emphasizing environmental and dietary factors. He especially recommended whole barley, the staple in ancient Greece and the Mediterranean world, supplemented with wheat and other grains and their products, aiong with simple, safe compresses made of grains, vegetables, and plants that could be prepared at home.

In his lectures and essays, Hippocrates focused on the energetics of food. In *Tradition in Medicine,* he explained: "I know too that the body is affected differently by bread according to the manner in which it is prepared. It differs according as it is made from pure flour or meal with bran, whether it is prepared from winnowed or unwinnowed wheat, whether it is mixed with much water or little, whether well mixed or poorly mixed, overbaked or underbaked, and countless other points besides. The same is true of the preparation of barley meal. The influence of each process is considerable and each has a totally different effect from another. How can anyone who has not considered such matters and come to understand them possibly know anything of the diseases that afflict mankind? Each one of the substances of a man's diet acts upon his body and changes it in some way and upon these changes his whole life depends . . . "

For many cases of illness, he recommended softly prepared barley (barley porridge or gruel), several times a day. He also utilized salt packs, baked millet compresses, and other applications to be placed on different parts of the body to promote circulation and provide comfort.

Source: *Hippocratic Writings*, G. E. R. Lloyd, editor, J. Chadwick and W. N. Mann, translators (New York: Penguin Books, 1978).

2. The Yellow Emperor's Classic

The *Yellow Emperor's Classic of Internal Medicine* (the *Nei Ching*) recommends whole cereal grains, especially millet and brown rice, as principal food. One of the world's oldest medical books, the Chinese text dates in written form to the third century B.C. but is believed to go back several thousand years earlier. The major source of theory and practice for Far Eastern medicine, the *Yellow Emperor's Classic* recommends a balanced diet to promote health and long life and to prevent and relieve serious disease.

"The Yellow Emperor once addressed Tien Shih, the divinely inspired teacher: I have heard that in ancient times the people lived to be over 100 years, and yet they remained active and did not become decrepit in their activities. But nowadays people reach only half that age and yet become decrepit and failing. Is it because the world changes from generation to generation? Or is it because mankind has become negligent of the laws of nature?

"Ch'i Po answered: In ancient times those people who understood the Tao patterned their lives according to Yin and Yang. And so they lived in harmony.

"There was temperance in eating and drinking. Their hours of rising and retiring were regular, and their lives were not disorderly and wild. By these means the ancients kept their bodies united with their souls, so as to fulfill their allotted span completely, measuring unto a hundred years and more before they passed away."

For serious illness, Ch'i Po relates, people treated disease "by cereal soups to be drunk for ten days." He particularly emphasizes the value of whole brown rice for nourishment and energy.

Modern medicine in China is confirming many of these recommendations. For example, Shi Zhaoqi, director of the Department of Proctology at Guanganmen Hospital, stated that hemorrhoids and their cause are mentioned in *The Yellow Emperor's Classic*, "In the text the disease was described as being caused by 'a disorder of the arteries and veins,' which is not unlike the modern diagnosis of 'pathogenic dilation of the blood vessels.'" Shi then used principles in the text and in T'ang Dynasty manuals (dating to the 7th century) to devise a dietary-based remedy.

Sources: Ilza Veith, translator, *The Yellow Emperor's Classic of Internal Medicine* (Berkeley: University of California Press, 1972); Henry C. Lu, translator, *A Complete Translation of Nei Ching and Nan Ching*, (Vancouver: The Academy of Oriental Heritage, 1978), and "Traditional Chinese Medicine Making Its Mark on the World," *Beijing Review*, May 19, 1986.

3. Book of Daniel

During the Babylonian Captivity, King Nebuchadnezzar commanded several of the most gifted young men of Israel to be brought to court to enter government service. The king instructed Malasar, the master of his household, to feed Daniel and his three companions the best meat and wine from the royal table. The Israelites, however, refused the rich food and instead asked for the simple grain-and-vegetable quality food they were accustomed to. The steward replied that he could lose his head if the king saw Daniel and his friends undernourished in comparison to the young Babylonians their age also in training for administrative service.

Daniel replied: "Submit us to this test for ten days. Give us only pulses [grains, seeds, and small beans] to eat and water to drink; then compare our looks with those of the young men who have lived on the food assigned by the king, and be guided in your treatment of us by what you see." At the end of ten days, Daniel and his friends were healthier and better nourished than the Babylonians and "the guard took away the assignment of food and the wine they were to drink, and gave them only the vegetables. And to these children God gave knowledge and understanding also of all visions and dreams."

Source: *Book of Daniel* 1:8-17.

4. Traditional Indian Medicine

The *Upanishads*, or early Forest Teachings in India, extol food as the essence of physical, mental, and spiritual development. The *Taittiriya Upanishad*, for example, states: "From food are born all creatures; they live upon food, they are dissolved in food. Food is the chief of all things, the universal medicine."

The *Caraka Samhita*, the principal text of Ayurveda, the traditional medicine of India, dates to the 1st or 2nd century A.D. It also emphasizes the central importance of diet in personal health and development of humanity.

"The use of beneficial food is the only cause of growth of a person, while the use of food that is injurious is the cause of disease."

"It is in consequence of this deterioration [in diet] that there took place a corresponding deterioration in the sap, purity, taste, potency, post-digestive effect and quality of herbs. In this manner, righteousness dwindles in each succeeding age by one quarter and the proto-elements too suffer deterioration, till eventually the world comes to dissolution."

Sources: Shree Purohit Swami and W. B. Yeats, translators, *The Upanishads* (London: Faber and Faber, 1937) and Ram K. Sharma and V.B. Dash, translators, *Caraka Samhita* (New York: Auromere, 1983).

5. Buddhist Medicine

Siddartha Gautama, the historical Buddha, attained universal understanding while eating brown rice and meditating under a tree in north India. In his teaching, he emphasized the psychological and medicinal value of a diet that avoided extremes. Eating brown rice, especially softly prepared rice, he said, gives many healthful blessings:

It confers ten things on him:

Life and beauty, ease and strength;
It dispels hunger, thirst, and wind.
It cleanses the bladder, it digests food;
This medicine is praised by the Well-Farer.

Source: I. B. Horner, translator, *The Book of the Discipline (Vinaya-pitaka)*, Vol. IV (London: 1951), p. 302.

6. Middle Eastern Medicine

The *Qu'ran* proclaims, "Let man examine his food," and has many passages upholding the beneficial value of wheat, barley, and other whole cereal grains. Islamic medicine developed a comprehensive approach synthesizing Hippocratic teachings from Greece and traditional Arabic folk remedies. Dietary recommendations formed the core of the medical system taught by Ibn Sina (Avicenna), a famous medieval physician, and his treatise on healing, *The Canon of Medicine*, served as the chief medical text in both Europe and Arabia until the beginning of modern times. Food continues to play a central role in Islamic medicine. "*Tibbi*, nutrition, is based on the concept that for each food, whether it is fruit, vegetable or meat, there is an energy, essence or state of quality that can be identified and formulated," explains Dr. Muhammad Salim Khan. "This enables the physician to express the essence of food in a holistic manner and context."

Moses Maimonides, the 12th century Jewish physician, upheld whole grain bread as the perfect food: "The bread should be made of coarse flour; that is to say, the husk should not be removed and the bran should not be refined by sifting. It should be well raised and noticeably salty. It should be well worked during kneading and should be baked in the oven. This is the bread that to the physician is properly prepared; it is the best of foods."

Sources: Muhammad Salim Khan, *Islamic Medicine* (London: Routledge & Kegan Paul, 1986) and Moses Maimonides, *Two Treatises on the Regimen of Health* (Philadelphia: American Philosophical Society, 1964).

7. Luigi Cornaro

In 1558 Luigi Cornaro, a Venetian-born architect and counselor, wrote an essay on health and diet describing how he suffered from a terminal stomach disorder in middle-age which he overcame by adopting a grain-based diet and avoiding certain kinds of animal food, raw salads, fruit, pastries, and sweets. Stating that we cannot partake of a "more natural food" than plain dark bread, Cornaro lived to age 102 and his book became one of the most influential books on health and diet during the Renaissance.

Source: Luigi Cornaro, *The Art of Living Long* (Milwaukee: William F. Butler, 1935).

8. Ekiken Kaibara

In 1713 Japanese physician Ekiken Kaibara recommended a balanced diet to protect against chronic disease. "A person should prefer light, simple meals. One must not eat a lot of heavy, greasy, rich food. One should also avoid uncooked, chilled, or hard food. . . . Of everything one eats and drinks, the most important thing is rice, which must be eaten in ample amounts to ensure proper nutrition . . . . Bean paste has a soft quality and is good for the stomach and intestines."

Source: Ekiken Kaibara, *Yojokun: Japanese Secret of Good Health* (Tokyo: Tokuma Shoten, 1974).

6. Christolph Von Hufeland

Christoph Von Hufeland, M.D., an eighteenth century German philosopher, professor of medicine, and physician to Goethe, recommended a simple grain-and-vegetable diet with thorough chewing, warned of the health hazards of meat and sugar, and promoted breastfeeding, exercise, and self-healing. "The more a man follows Nature, and is obedient to her laws, the longer he will live; the further he deviates from these the shorter will be his existence," he noted in his book *Macrobiotics, or the Art of Prolonging Life.* "The healing power of nature must, above all things, be supported from the beginning, because it is the principal means which lies in ourselves for rendering the causes of disease ineffectual. This may be done chiefly by not accustoming the body at first too much to artificial assistance; otherwise Nature will be so used that she will depend on foreign aid, and at length lose altogether the power of assisting herself."

In regard to dietary practice, he observed, "Rich and nourishing food, and an immoderate use of flesh, do not prolong life. Instances of the greatest age are to be found among men who from their youth lived principally on vegetables, and who perhaps never tasted flesh."

In regard to lifestyle, he stated, "[T]he degree of civilization, luxury, refinement, and deviation from nature, in which we at present live, by so highly exalting our intensive life, tends also to shorten, in the same proportion, our existence."

Source: C. W. Hufeland, M.D., *Macrobiotics or the Art of Prolonging Life,* 1796.

7. Namboku Mizuno

Namboku Mizuno, an 18th century Japanese physiognomist, challenged the way that visual diagnosis and fortune-telling had been practiced in the Far East for many centuries. He taught that fortune, health, and wealth are not fixed by heaven but are governed by diet, lifestyle, and environment. No matter how starcrossed one's face or palm, he held that a person could control his or her destiny by observing a natural way of living, especially by limiting the intake of food. During his lifetime, he gave advice to thousands of parents and children, merchants and priests, geisha and samurai, intellectuals and sumo wrestlers, criminals and the mentally ill who were seeking advice on their worldly and spiritual fate. In his book on diet, health, and life-extention, he observed, "One who understands heaven and earth's grace will not waste anything and knows his action brings in happiness and longevity according to the order of heaven. Therefore, he even enjoys more being humble and frugal, and then his mind will become peaceful, and automatically the *ki* of his personality will be nourished. He will naturally create great *ki* energy. But someone who loves sake, meat, and rich food will spoil his mind and body, and automatically he will destroy such great *ki* energy, and his life will be short." He recommended a simple grain-and-vegetable diet for usual good health and soft rice for sickness.

Source: Michio and Aveline Kushi and Alex Jack, translators, *Food Governs Your Destiny: The Teachings of Namboku Mizuno* (Tokyo and New York: Japan Publications, 1991).

8. Walking John Stuart

John Stuart, an adventurous Englishman who set off on various hikes, expeditions, and pilgrimages across Europe and Asia, earned the nickname "Walking John." In the course of his travels, he observed the health and diets of the countries through which he passed. "I have observed among nations whose aliment is vegetables and water that disease and medicine are equally unknown," he noted, "while those whose ailment is flesh and fermented liquor are constantly afflicted with disease and with medicine more dangerous than disease itself."

Source: John Stuart, *Journals*, 1790.

9. Sagen Ishizuka

At the end of the 19th century, Japanese physician and philosopher Sagen Ishizuka, M.D., published the results of many years' research and study, outlining a broad theory of human physiology, food, health, sickness and medicine based on the dynamic balance between sodium and potassium in the environment and diet. On the basis of his own work as a military doctor in China and general practitioner in Japan, as well as readings in anthropology, he concluded that whole cereal grains contained the ideal balance of nutrients and should form the foundation of the human diet, supplemented with beans, vegetables, seeds and nuts, and a small amount of fish or game depending on the climate, region, and season of the year. In Tokyo, he set up a free clinic and was known as "Dr. Daikon" and "Dr. Miso Soup." He helped thousands of people recover from tuberculosis, diptheria, and other modern diseases that had entered Japan with the modern diet.

Sources: Sagen Ishizuka, *Kagakuteki Shoku-Yo (A Chemical Nutritional Theory of Long Life)*, 1897 (Tokyo: Nippon C.I., 1975), and *Shokumotsu Yojoho: Ichimei Kagakuteki Shoku-Yo Tai Shin Ron (A Method for Nourishing Life Through Food: A Unique Chemical Food-Nourishment Theory of Body and Mind)*, 1898 (Tokyo: Nippon C.I., 1974).

10. Hunza Diet

From 1904 to 1911 British surgeon Robert McCarrison traveled in the Hunza, a remote Himalayan kingdom in the then Northwest Territory of India. There he was astonished to discover a completely healthy culture in which the infectious and degenerative diseases of modern civilization, including colonial India, were unknown. "I never saw a case of asthenic dyspepsia, of gastric or duodenal ulcer, of appendicitis, of mucous colitis, or of cancer," he informed his medical colleagues. McCarrison theorized that the unusual health and longevity of the Hunza people were due primarily to their daily diet of whole-wheat chapatis, barley, and maize, supplemented by leafy green vegetables, beans and legumes, apricots, and a small amount of animal food. The Hunzas did not eat refined white rice, sugar, black tea, or spices as did most of the Indian population. In 1927 as Director of Nutritional Reseach in India, Dr. McCarrison discovered that rats fed the modern, refined diet of Bengal and Madras contracted cysts, abscesses, heart disease, and cancer of the stomach, while those fed the Hunza whole-grain diet remained healthy and free of all disease.

Sources: Robert McCarrison, M.D., "Faulty Food in Relation to Gastro-Intestinal Disorder," *Journal of the American Medical Association* 78:1-8, 1922, and G. T. Wrench, M.D., *The Wheel of Health* (London: O. W. Daniel, 1938).

11. Dr. Albert Schweitzer

Looking back over four decades of medical work in French Equatorial Africa, Dr. Albert Schweitzer reported that he had never had any cancer cases in his hospital and that its occurrence among the African people was very rare. He attributed the rise of degenerative diseases to the importation of European foods including condensed milk, canned butter, meat and fish preserves, white bread, and especially refined salt. "It is obvious to connect the fact of increase of cancer with the increased use of salt by the natives. In former years there was only available the little salt extracted from the ocean."

Source: Albert Schweitzer, M.D., *Briefe aus dem Lambarenespital*, 1954.

12. George Ohsawa

In 1913, Yukikazu Sakurazawa, later known as George Ohsawa, healed himself of terminal pulmonary tuberculosis after reading a book on health and diet by Sagen Ishizuka. Over the next fifty years, Ohsawa devoted his life to spreading macrobiotics and guiding thousands of people to health and happiness. Among the many medical and scientific experiments he conducted, in 1941 he oversaw the treatment of twenty-three sick and wounded soldiers at a military recuperation center in Tokyo. All medications were stopped, and the soldiers were fed brown rice and vegetables. Wounds and infections were treated with salt water only. After one month, all the men had made progress physically and their morale was higher. In another experiment, while visiting Dr. Schweitzer in Africa, George Ohsawa deliberately contracted tropical ulcers — an invariably fatal disease — in order to show that it could be reversed by dietary methods. Taking plenty of salt and umeboshi (salted plums), he completely recovered from this affliction which he said was spreading among the African people who were eating sugar, refined foods, and excessive fruits and fungi.

In *The Book of Judgment*, Ohsawa observed: "To eat is to live. To live is to give, as shown in our logarithmic spiral. All beings live to give their products and the whole of their life, to become a bit higher being. Many men do not know that *vivere parvo* [voluntary poverty] is the only way to enter into the country of eternal happiness." Among the case histories he presented are men and women who used a balanced diet to overcome polio, asthma, leprosy, epilepsy, and schizophrenia. In a typical case (classified as "Foolhardiness"), he noted: "Mr. X, a clerk in a big industrial company in Calcutta, had lost his job because he became insane. His oldest brother had brought him to me from afar, hoping that my dietetic method would cure him.

"The patient did not speak. He sat night and day in a corner of his brother's house. He would neither eat nor drink. But occasionally he would run away and he would then wander through the big strange city for days. His brother always had great difficulty in finding him.

"'This is an intoxication, probably from white sugar,' I said. Indeed, he was the supervisor in a great sugar warehouse. All his colleagues were stealing and selling sugar, but being more honest, he was satisfied with taking only as much sugar as he could eat.

"Once the ultimate cause was known, healing was easy. He was cured in five weeks. Had he had the usual psychiatric treatment, he would very likely have been confined in a hospital, perhaps for the remainder of his life."

Sources: George Ohsawa, *Hitotsu no Hokuku: Aru Byoin ni okeru Jikken no Kokoku* (*A Report of a Hospital Experiment*) 1941 (Tokyo: Nippon C.I., 1976); *The Book of Judgment* (Oroville, Ca.: George Ohsawa Macrobiotic Foundation, 1966); *Macrobiotics — The Way of Healing* (G.O.M.F., 1985).

13. Weston Price

For many years dental surgeon Weston Price performed field-work among the Indians of North America, the Inuit, the Polynesians, and the Australian Aborigines and reported no trace of cancer, heart disease, and other degenerative illnesses among those cultures and communities following traditional ways of eating. He noted that the diseases of modern civilization appeared only following the introduction of white flour, white rice, sugar, canned food, and other articles of modern diet.

Source: Weston Price, D.D.S., *Nutrition and Physical Degeneration* (Santa Monica: Price-Pottenger Nutritional Foundation, 1945).

14. The Paleolithic Diet

• The traditional diet of humanity has consisted of foods of primarily vegetable quality rather than meat and other animal food as popularly believed. "Recent investigations into the dietary habits of prehistoric peoples and their primate predecessors suggest that heavy meat-eating by modern affluent societies may be exceeding the biological capacities evolution built into the human body. The result may be a host of diet-related health problems, such as diabetes, obesity, high blood pressure, coronary heart disease, and some cancers. The studies challenge the notion that human beings evolved as aggressive hunting animals who depended primarily upon meat for survival. The new view — coming from findings in such fields as archaeology, anthropology, primatology, and comparative anatomy — instead portrays early humans and their forebears more as herbivores than carnivores. According to these studies, the prehistoric table for at least the last million and a half years was probably set with three times more plant than animal foods, the reverse of what the average American currently eats."

Source: Jane E. Brody, "Research Yields Surprises About Early Human Diets," *New York Times*, Science Section, May 15, 1979.

• Anthropologists reported that the traditional diet of paleolithic times, including wild grains, roots, beans, nuts, tubers, and fruits, as well as wild game, appeared to be protective against cancer, heart disease, and other diseases. "Differences between the dietary patterns of our remote ancestors and the patterns now prevalent in

Paleolithic and Modern Dietary Composition			
	Paleolithic Diet	**Standard American Diet**	**Current Dietary Recommendations**
Dietary Energy (%)			
Protein	33	12	12
Carbohydrate	46	46	58
Fat	21	42	30
Poly/Sat Lipid Ratio	1.41	0.44	1
Fiber (g)	100-150	19.7	30-60
Sodium (mg)	690	2300-6900	1000-3300
Calcium (mg)	1500-2000	740	800-1500
Ascorbic Acid (mg)	440	90	60
Source: New England Journal of Medicine, 1985			

industrialized countries appear to have important implications for health, and the specific pattern of nutritional disease is a function of the stage of civilization." Although some ancient societies ate more animal food than today, the amount and type of fat consumed was very different. Modern domesticated animals contain about eight to ten times more fat than their wild counterparts, and wild game contains over five times more polyunsaturated fat per gram than is found in domestic livestock which is highly saturated in quality. "The diet of our remote ancestors may be a reference standard for modern human nutrition and a model for defense against certain 'diseases of civilization,'" the researchers concluded.

Source: S. B. Eaton and M. Konner, "Paleolithic Nutrition," *New England Journal of Medicine* 313:283-89, 1985.

• The few Stone Age cultures remaining in the world today consume primarily vegetable-quality food. Scientists who studied fifty-eight contemporary hunter-gatherer societies found that their diets contained from 50 to 70 percent complex carbohydrates from plant sources. Animal food comprised 25 to 30 percent of the total volume, and none of the tribes consumed milk, sugar, alcohol, or salt added at the meal.

Source: H. C. Trowell and D. P. Burkitt, *Western Diseases: Their Emergence and Prevention* (Cambridge, Mass.: Harvard University Press, 1981), p. 15.

15. Native American Diet

The native peoples of North America traditionally ate a diet centered around corn, beans, and squash and used food as medicine. A gruel of parched cornmeal was commonly used for fever and other sicknesses. Many Indians avoided the use of salt and fresh meat during illness. Nursing mothers took a light soup or broth made of flint corn during the first three days after delivery in order to produce nourishing milk for their babies.

Source: Virgil J. Vogel, *American Indian Medicine* (Norman, Ok.: University of Oklahoma Press, 1970).

16. Tarahumara Indians

The Tarahumara Indians are the healthiest native community in North America. The Tarahumaras live in the Sierra Madre Occidental Mountains in north central Mexico and eat a traditional diet of corn, beans, and squash. Meat is seldom eaten, and eggs are taken only occasionally. The 50,000 Tarahumaras use no mechanical energy in farming, travel only by foot, and engage in marathon kickball competitions. Researchers who have studied this native culture report that high blood pressure and obesity are absent and death from heart and other degenerative diseases are unknown.

Source: W. E. Connor, "The Plasma Lipids, Lipoproteins, and Diet of the Tarahumara Indians of Mexico," *American Journal of Clinical Nutrition* 31: 1131-42, 1978.

17. African Diet

Medical researchers in Senegal produced a cough syrup from gueira, a native plant that is as effective as codeine-based medicines imported from Europe. They also made a laxative from the lam plant. At the World Health Organization's (W.H.O.) Collaborating Center of Traditional Medicine at the University of Illinois, these and other medicinal plants from Africa and around the world are available in a computer database.

Source: Thomas Land, "Folk Cures Gain Respect and Save Money," *Toward Freedom*, April/May, 1991, pp. 17-18.

Food Changes 1910-1976			
Per capita annual consumption in pounds unless noted otherwise			
Category	1910	1976	Change
Grains	**294**	**144**	**-51%**
Wheat	214	112	-48%
Corn	51.1	7.7	-85%
Rice	7.2	7.2	none
Barley	3.5	1.2	-66%
Oats	3.5	3.5	none
Vegetables	**188**	**144.5**	**-23%**
Cabbage	23.2 (1920)	8.3	-64%
Fresh Potato	80.4	48.3	-40%
Frozen Potato	6.6 (1960)	36.8	+457
Tomato Products	5.0 (1920)	22.4	+348
Canned Vegetables	12.6 (1920)	53.0	+320
Frozen Vegetables	.57 (1940)	9.9	+1,650
Fresh Fruit	**123**	**82.0**	**-33%**
Processed Fruit	20.5	134.6	+556
Frozen Citrus	1.0 (1948)	117.0	+11,600
Frozen Foods	3.1 (1940)	88.8	+2,764
Meat	**136.2**	**165.2**	**+21%**
Beef	55.5	95.4	+72%
Poultry	**18.0**	**52.9**	**+194%**
Eggs	**305 whole**	**276 whole**	**-10%**
Fish	**11.4**	**13.7**	**+20%**
Dairy	**320.2**	**354.3**	**+11%**
Whole Milk	29.3 gal.	21.5 gal.	-27%
Low Fat Milk	6.8 gal.	10.6 gal.	+56%
Cheese	4.9	20.7	+322%
Ice Cream	1.9	18.1	+852%
Frozen Dairy	3.4	50.2	+1,376%
Sweeteners	**89.0**	**134.6**	**+51%**
Corn Syrup	3.8	32.7	+761%
Sugar	73.7 (1909)	94.8	+29%
Soft Drinks	1.1 gal.	30.8 gal.	+2,638%
Source: U.S.D.A.			

2

Modern Dietary Guidelines

To future generations, Dietary Goals for the United States *may be regarded as the Magna Carta of humanity's return to a healthier way of eating. After two years of public hearings during which vegetarian and macrobiotic teachers, nutritionists, school teachers, correction officials, parents, and others were allowed to present their experience of the relation of diet and degenerative disease, the Senate Select Committee on Nutrition and Human Needs issued a report in 1977 linking the modern diet with six of the leading causes of death including heart disease and cancer. Until this time, the government, along with most of the scientific and medical community, had given uncritical support to the modern diet high in meat and other animal food, sugar, refined flour, highly processed foods, and foods grown or treated with chemicals, additives, and other artificial ingredients. The McGovern Report, as it was also known after its chairman Senator George McGovern, sent shock waves through the schools, hospitals, farms, and research centers around the world. Within the next several years, all major scientific and medical associations issued similar reports.*

18. *Dietary Goals*

Summarizing its conclusions on the nation's way of eating, health, and future direction, *Dietary Goals for the United States* stated: "During this century, the composition of the average diet in the United States has changed radically. Complex carbohydrates —

fruit, vegetables, and grain products — which were the mainstay of the diet, now play a minority role. At the same time, fat and sugar consumption have risen to the point where these two dietary elements alone now comprise at least 60 percent of total calorie intake, up from 50 percent in the early 1900s. In the view of doctors and nutritionists consulted by the Select Committee, these and other changes in the diet amount to a wave of malnutrition — of both over- and under-consumption — that may be as profoundly damaging to the Nation's health as the widespread contagious diseases of the early part of this century. The over-consumption of fat, generally, and saturated fat in particular, as well as cholesterol, sugar, salt, and alcohol have been related to six of the leading causes of death: Heart disease, cancer, cerebrovascular diseases, diabetes, arteriosclerosis, and cirrhosis of the liver."

The report listed six dietary goals:

1. Increase carbohydrate consumption to account for 55 to 60 percent of the energy (caloric) intake.

2. Reduce overall fat consumption from approximately 40 to 30 percent of energy intake.

3. Reduce saturated fat consumption to account for about 10 percent of total energy intake; and balance with polyunsaturated and monounsaturated fats, which should account for about 10 percent of energy intake each.

4. Reduce cholesterol consumption to about 300 mg. a day.

5. Reduce sugar consumption by almost 40 percent to account for about 15 percent of total energy intake.

6. Reduce salt consumption by about 50 to 85 percent to approximately 3 grams a day.

The goals suggest the following changes in food selection and preparation:

1. Increase consumption of fruits and vegetables and whole grains.

2. Decrease consumption of meat and increase consumption of poultry and fish.

3. Decrease consumption of foods high in fat and partially substitute polyunsaturated fat for saturated fat.

4. Substitute non-fat milk for whole milk.

5. Decrease consumption of butterfat, eggs, and other high cholesterol sources.

6. Decrease consumption of sugar and foods that are high in

Nutritional Comparisons			
	Current American Diet	U.S. Dietary Goals	Macrobiotic Diet
Fat Intake	42	30	15
Saturated	16	10	2
Monounsaturated	19	10	8
Polyunsaturated	7	10	5
Protein	12	12	12
Carbohydrate	46	58	73
Complex	28	48	73
Refined	18	10	0

Sources: *U.S. Dietary Goals, 1977 and The Book of Macrobiotics, 1978*

sugar content.

7. Decrease consumption of salt and foods high in salt content.

Source: Select Committee on Nutrition and Human Needs, U.S. Senate, *Dietary Goals for the United States* (Washington, D.C.: U.S. Government Printing Office, 1977).

19. *Surgeon-General's Report*

In 1979 the U.S. Surgeon General issued a report that suggested degenerative disease could be relieved as well as prevented by dietary means and called for substantial increases in the consumption of whole grains, vegetables, and fresh fruit and reductions in meat, eggs, dairy food, sugar, and other processed foods. The report stated: "A good case can be made for the role of high intake of cholesterol and saturated fat, usually of animal origin, in producing high blood cholesterol levels which are associated with atherosclerosis and cardiovascular diseases.

"Animal studies have shown that reducing serum cholesterol can slow down and even reverse the atherosclerotic process.

"And, in man, certain studies have shown that people in countries where diets are low in saturated fats and cholesterol have lower average serum cholesterol levels and fewer heart attacks; and that Americans who habitually eat less fat-rich diets (vegetarians [macrobiotics] and Seventh Day Adventists, for example) have less heart disease than other Americans; and that atherosclerotic plaques in certain arteries may be reversed by cholesterol-lowering diets."

The report concluded that while individual nutritional standards would be hard to establish because of varying conditions and personal needs, Americans would probably be healthier, as a whole, if they consumed:

• Only sufficient calories to meet body needs and maintain desirable weight (fewer calories if overweight).

• Less salt.

• Less sugar.

• Relatively more complex carbohydrates such as whole grains, cereals, fruits and vegetables.

• Relatively more fish, poultry, legumes (e.g., beans, peas, peanuts) and less red meat.

The Surgeon-General further warned against the processing of modern foods. "The American food supply has changed so that more than half of our diet now consists of processed foods rather than fresh agricultural produce. . . . Increased attention therefore also needs to be paid to the nutritional qualities of processed food."

Source: *Healthy People: The Surgeon General's Report on Health Promotion and Disease Prevention* (Washington, D.C.: Government Printing Office, 1979).

20. American Heart Association

Since the 1960s, the American Heart Association has cited faulty diet as the main cause of cardiovascular disease and continually revised its dietary guidelines in the direction of more whole, unprocessed foods. "Habitual excesses in eating habits — especially of fats, salt, and possibly sugar — are high on the list of controllable factors that have been linked to cardiovascular disease. . . . it is recommended that the proportion of fat to the total caloric intake be kept to somewhere between 30 and 35 percent, and that vegetable (polyunsaturated) fat be substituted for that from animal sources as an important means of lessening the risk of atherosclerosis and coronary disease. . . . Most people in the United States consume more protein than they need. To lessen the risk of cardiovascular disease, the balance should be shifted in favor of more complex carbohydrates, such as are found in fresh fruits and vegetables. On the other hand, overindulgence in the chemically simpler sugars, in the form of desserts, soft drinks, and snack foods, is to be avoided.... "

The 1985 American Heart Association Diet stated that fat intake could be reduced even lower than 30 percent. The list of recommended daily foods included a wide range of vegetables and fruits, including broccoli, cabbage, mustard greens, kale, collards, carrots, pumpkins, and winter squash; breads, cereals, pasta, and starchy vegetables including whole-grain bread and brown rice; low-fat meat and poultry, fish and seafood, nuts, dried beans, peas, and other meatless main entries including tofu; and vegetable-quality fats and oils. The list of foods to avoid included whole milk, most cheeses, ice cream, and other high-fat dairy products; eggs (maximum 2 per week) and foods prepared with eggs; red-meat (except for lean cuts), cured meat, and organ meats; butter and other animal-quality fats and hydrogenated fats and oils; sugary desserts, store-bought desserts and mixes, and highly processed snacks.

Source: *The American Heart Association Heartbook* (New York: Dutton, 1980), pp. 65-66 and "The American Heart Association Diet" (Dallas: American Heart Association, 1985).

21. *Diet, Nutrition, and Cancer*

In 1982 the National Academy of Sciences issued *Diet, Nutrition, and Cancer*, a 472-page report in which the modern diet high in saturated fat, animal protein, sugar, and chemical additives was associated with a majority of cancers, including malignancies of the breast, colon, prostate, uterus, stomach, lung, and esophagus. The panel reviewed hundreds of current medical studies associating long-term eating patterns with the development of of 30 to 40 percent of cancers in men and 60 percent in women. "Just as it was once difficult for investigators to recognize that a symptom complex could be caused by the lack of a nutrient," the panel noted, "so until recently has it been difficult for scientists to recognize that certain pathological conditions might result from an abundant and apparently normal diet." The report issued interim dietary guidelines calling for substantial decreases in meat, poultry, egg, dairy, and refined carbohydrate consumption and increased consumption of whole cereal grains, vegetables and fruits:

1. There is sufficient evidence that high fat consumption is linked to increased incidence of certain cancers (notably breast and colon cancer) and that low fat intake is associated with a lower incidence of these cancers. The committee recommends that the consumption of both saturated and unsaturated fats be reduced in the average U.S. diet. An appropriate and practical target is to reduce the intake of fat from its present level (approximately 40 percent) to 30 percent of total calories in the diet. The scientific data do not provide a strong basis for establishing fat intake at precisely 30 percent of total calories. Indeed, the data could be used to justify an even greater reduction. However, in the judgment of the committee, the suggested reduction (i.e., one-quarter of the fat intake) is a moderate and practical target, and is likely to be beneficial.

2. The committee emphasizes the importance of including fruits, vegetables, and whole grain cereal products in the daily diet. In epidemiological studies, frequent consumption of these foods has been inversely correlated with the incidence of various cancers. Results of laboratory experiments have supported these findings in tests of individual nutritive and nonnutritive constituents of fruits (especially citrus fruits) and vegetables (especially carotene-rich and cruciferous vegetables).

These recommendations apply only to foods as sources of nutrients — not to dietary supplements of individual nutrients. The vast literature examined in this report focuses on the relationship between the consumption of foods and the incidence of cancer in human populations. In contrast, there is very little information of the effects of various levels of individual nutrients on the risk of cancer in humans. Therefore, the committee is unable to predict the health effects of high and potentially toxic doses of isolated nutrients consumed in the form of supplements.

3. In some parts of the world, especially China, Japan, and Iceland, populations that frequently consumed salt-cured (including salt-pickled) or smoked foods have a greater incidence of cancers at some sites, especially the esophagus and the stomach. In addition, some methods of smoking and pickling foods seem to produce higher levels of polycyclic aromatic hydrocarbons and N-nitroso compounds. These compounds cause mutations in bacteria and cancer in animals and are suspected of being carcinogenic in humans. Therefore, the committee recommends that the consumption of food preserved by salt-curing (including salt-pickling) or smoking

be minimized.

4. Certain non-nutritive constituents of foods, whether naturally occurring or introduced inadvertently (as contaminants) during production, processing, and storage, pose a potential risk of cancer to humans. The committee recommends that efforts continued to be made to minimize contamination of foods with carcinogens from any source. Where such contaminants are unavoidable, permissible levels should continued to be established and the food supply monitored to assure that such levels are not exceeded. Furthermore, intentional additives (direct and indirect) should continue to be evaluated for carcinogenic activity before they are approved for use in the food supply.

5. The committee suggests that further efforts be made to identify mutagens in food and to expedite testing for their carcinogenicity. Where feasible and prudent, mutagens should be removed or their concentration minimized when this can be accomplished without jeopardizing the nutritive value of foods or introducing other potentially hazardous substances into the diet.

6. Excessive consumption of alcoholic beverages, particularly combined with cigarette smoking, has been associated with an increased risk of cancer of the upper gastrointestinal and respiratory tracts. Consumption of alcohol is also associated with other adverse health effects. Thus, the committee recommends that if alcoholic beverages are consumed, it be done in moderation.

The report noted in conclusion, "The dietary changes now underway appear to be reducing our dependence on foods from animal sources. It is likely that there will be continued reduction in fats from animal sources and an increasing dependence on vegetable and other plant products for protein supplies. Hence, diets may contain increasing amounts of vegetable products, some of which may be protective against cancer."

Source: National Academy of Sciences, *Diet, Nutrition, and Cancer* (Washington, D.C.: National Academy Press, 1982).

22. American Cancer Society

In 1984, the American Cancer Society issued dietary guidelines for the first time in respect to the cause and prevention of cancer: "There is now good reason to suspect that dietary habits contribute to human cancer, but it is important to understand that the interpretation of both human population (epidemiologic) and laboratory data is very complex, and as yet does not allow clear-cut conclusions. . . . Foods may have constituents that cause or promote cancer on the one hand or protect against it on the other. No concrete dietary advice can be given that will guarantee prevention of any specific human cancer. The American Cancer Society nonetheless believes that there is sufficient inferential information to make a series of interim recommendations about nutrition that, in the judgment of experts, are likely to provide some measure of reducing cancer risk . . .

Recommendations:

1. Avoid obesity.
2. Cut down on total fat intake.
3. Eat more high fiber foods, such as whole grain cereals, fruits and vegetables.
4. Include foods rich in vitamins A and C in the daily diet.
5. Include cruciferous vegetables, such as cabbage, broccoli, Brussels sprouts, kohlrabi, and cauliflower in the diet.
6. Be moderate in consumption of alcoholic beverages.
7. Be moderate in consumption of salt-cured, smoked, and nitrite-cured foods.

Source: *Nutrition and Cancer: Cause and Prevention* (New York: American Cancer Society, 1984).

23. American Medical Association

In its newly revised dietary guidelines, the American Medical Association recommended:

1. Eat meat no more than once a day, and choose fish or poultry over red-meat.
2. Bake or broil food rather than frying it and use polyunsaturated oils rather than butter, lard, or margarine.
3. Cut down on salt, MSG, and other flavorings high in sodium.
4. Eat more fiber including whole grain cereals, leafy green vegetables, and fruit.
5. Eat no more than four eggs a week.
6. For dessert or a snack, eat fruit rather than baked goods.

In a review of special diets, the nation's major medical association advised: "In the macrobiotic diet foods fall into two main groups, known as yin and yang (based on an Eastern principle of opposites), depending on where they have been grown, their texture, color, and composition. The general principle behind this diet is that foods biologically furthest away from us are better for us. Cereals, therefore, form the basis of the diet and fish is preferred to meat. Although fresh foods free of additives are preferred, no food is actually prohibited, in the belief that a craving for any food may refect a genuine bodily need. In general, the macrobiotic diet is a healthful way of eating. However, extreme adherents of macrobiotics restrict fluid intake, and this could be harmful to health."

Source: *The American Medical Association Family Medical Guide,* (New York: Random House, 1987).

24. Canadian Dietary Guidelines

In 1977 the Canadian Department of National Health and Welfare issued dietary recommendations as follows:

• The consumption of a nutritionally adequate diet, as outlined in Canada's *Food Guide.*

• A reduction in the proportion of fat in the diet to 35 percent of the total energy intake. A source of polyunsaturated fatty acid (linoleic acid) should be included in the diet.

• The consumption of a diet that emphasizes whole-grain products and fruits and vegetables and minimizes alcohol, salt, and refined sugars.

• The prevention and control of obesity through a reduction in excess consumption of food and an increase in physical activity. Precautions should be taken that no deficiency of vitamins and minerals occurs when the total energy intake is reduced.

Source: "Nutrition Recommendations for Canadians," *Canadian Medical Association Journal* 120(10):1241-42, 1979.

25. British Dietary Guidelines

In 1983 the National Advisory Committee on Nutritional Education (N.A.C.N.E.) presented dietary goals for the United Kingdom. The *Lancet,* the U.K.'s chief medical journal, summarized the goals as follows:

"The long-term dietary goals set out in the report of the N.A.C.N.E. working party propose substantial reductions in the national consumption of fat (25 percent for total and 40 percent for saturated fat), sugar (50 percent), and salt (25 percent), and a rise in consumption of dietary fibre (50 percent). A reduction in alcohol consumption is also recommended. . . .

"The British diet, in common with nearly all national diets, is constantly changing. Until about 200 years ago, sucrose was eaten in very small amounts and only by the affluent. The intake proposed by the N.A.C.N.E. working party corresponds to that in 1870-74. For the mass of the population, total fat consumption was below 30 percent of total energy until well into this century. Those who doubt the practicality of change may overlook the substantial changes in the British diet since 1945 and even in the past 10 or 15 years, towards a higher level of processing and the introduction of many new foods of which a large number are not British in origin (e.g., hamburgers, yogurt, pasta)."

Source: "Implementing the N.A.C.N.E. Report," *Lancet* 2:1151-56, 1983.

26. Japanese Dietary Guidelines

The Panel on Nutrition and Prevention of Diseases in Japan issued dietary recommendations in 1983 calling for:
* Avoidance of excess total fat.
* Consumption of fresh fruits and vegetables, especially green and yellow vegetables, oranges, carotene, and fungi.
* Increased consumption of unrefined whole grain cereals, seaweed, and fiber-rich legumes.
* Restricted salt intake.
* Avoidance of hot drinks and burned food.
* Adoption of a varied diet and chewing food well.

In 1985 the Japanese Ministry of Health and Welfare issued dietary recommendations calling for:
* Reduction of total fat to 20 to 25 percent of calories.
* Reduction in saturated fat intake.
* Increased use of vegetable and fish oil.
* Restriction of salt consumption to 10 grams or less a day.
* Adoption of a varied diet (at least 30 foods daily).
* Home cooking.
* Creation of a pleasant eating environment.

Sources: Panel on Nutrition and Prevention of Diseases, 1983, and "Dietary

Guidelines for Health Promotion," Vol. 29 (Health Promotion and Nutrition Division, Health Services Bureau, Japanese Ministry of Health and Welfare, Tokyo, 1985).

27. Diet and Health

Diet and Health, the National Academy of Science's landmark 749-page report on "The Implications for Reducing Chronic Disease Risk," called in 1989 for the nation to substantially reduce animal food consumption and increase intake of whole cereal grains, fresh vegetables, and fruits.

After a comprehensive review of the epidemiologic, clinical, and laboratory evidence, the panel's nineteen experts concluded that the modern diet influences the risk of several major chronic diseases including atherosclerotic cardiovascular diseases, hypertension, cancers of the esophagus, stomach, large bowel, breast, lung, and prostate, dental caries, chronic liver disease, obesity, and noninsulin-dependent diabetes mellitus.

Conversely, the researchers found that a diet characterized by plant foods is associated with a lower risk of coronary heart disease, cancers of the lung, colon, esophagus, and stomach, diabetes mellitus, diverticulosis, hypertension, and gallstone formation. The committee recommended that the intake of carbohydrates be increased to more than 55 percent of total calories, especially complex carbohydrates as found in whole cereal grains, legumes, breads, vegetables, and certain fruits. Regular consumption of green and yellow vegetables was also encouraged.

"The committee notes that several countries with dietary patterns similar to those recommended in this report have about half the U.S. rates for diet-associated cancers. This suggests that the committee's dietary recommendations could have a substantial impact on reducing the risk of cancer in the United States."

In a review of "Alternative Diets," the report noted: "[T]he U.S. population consumes relatively large amounts of meat and sugar, more refined than whole-grain products, and larger amounts of commercially processed than fresh foods. In contrast, most of the world's population today subsists on vegetarian or near-vegetarian diets for reasons that are economic, philosophical, religious, cultural, or ecological. Indeed, humans appear to have subsisted for most of their history on near-vegetarian diets."

Vegetarian and Nonvegetarian Nutritive Value of Food Intake as a Percentage of the 1980 RDA*					
Diet	Number	Food Energy	Protein	Calcium	Iron
Vegetarian	464	83%	150%	104%	103%
Nonvegetarian	35,671	84%	165%	87%	102%
	Magnesium	Phosphorus	Vit. A	Thiamine	Riboflavin
Vegetarian	95%	146%	163%	117%	136%
Nonvegetarian	83%	136%	132%	113%	124%
	Performed Niacin	Vit. B6	Vit. B12	Vit. C	
Vegetarian	114%	76%	156%	176%	
Nonvegetarian	124%	75%	176%	147%	

*Average per individual per day (1977-78) measured as daily intake, % of RDA, for all sexes and ages except breast-fed infants, based on 3 consecutive days of dietary intake.

Reviewing current studies of vegetarians, the panel found that they "had lower intakes of protein, preformed niacin, and vitamin B_{12} than nonvegetarians, but that their average intakes of all three nutrients were above the RDAs. All other nutrients were, on average, at the same level or higher in vegetarian than in nonvegetarian diets." These included calcium, vitamin A, vitamin C, and magnesium. The committee also found that vegetarian females of reproductive age (nineteen to thirty-four) had comparable iron intakes as nonvegetarians and higher intakes of calcium, magnesium, phosphorus, vitamin A, riboflavin, vitamin B_{12}, vitamin C, vitamin B_6 and thiamine.

The dietary recommendations of the committee are as follows:

• Reduce total fat intake to 30 percent or less of calories. Reduce saturated fatty acid intake to less than 10 percent of calories and the intake of cholesterol to less than 300 mg daily. The intake of fat and cholesterol can be reduced by substituting fish, poultry without skin, lean meats, and low- or nonfat dairy products for fatty meats and whole-milk dairy products; by choosing more vegetables, fruits, cereals, and legumes; and by limiting oils, fats, egg yolks, and fried and other fatty foods.

• Every day eat five or more servings of a combination of vegetables and fruits, especially green and yellow vegetables and citrus fruits. Also, increase intake of starches and other complex carbohydrates by eating six or more daily servings of a combination of breads, cereals, and legumes.

• Maintain protein intake at moderate levels.

• Balance food intake and physical activity to maintain appropriate body weight.

• The committee does not recommend alcohol consumption. For those who drink alcoholic beverages, the committee recommends limiting consumption to the equivalent of less than 1 ounce of pure alcohol in a single day. This is the equivalent of two cans of beer, two small glasses of wine, or two average cocktails. Pregnant women should avoid alcoholic beverages.

• Limit total daily intake of salt (sodium choloride) to 6 grams or less. Limit the use of salt in cooking and avoid adding it to food at the table. Salty, highly processed salty, salt-preserved, and salt-pickled foods should be consumed sparingly.

• Maintain adequate calcium intake.

• Avoid taking dietary supplements in excess of the RDA in any one day.

• Maintain an optimal intake of fluoride, particularly during the years of primary and secondary tooth formation and growth.

Source: National Academy of Sciences, *Diet and Health: Implications for Reducing Chronic Disease Risk* (Washington, D.C.: National Academy Press) 1989.

28. *Dietary Guidelines for Americans*

In newly revised *Dietary Guidelines for Americans*, the U.S. Department of Agriculture and Department of Health and Human Services called for everyone to consume six to eleven servings of grains or grain products every day including whole-grain breads, cereals, pasta, and rice. (This constitutes about 40 percent of the daily diet.) Vegetables constituted the second biggest category of foods, with three to five servings, including dark green leafy and deep yellow vegetables, dry beans and peas, and starchy vegetables such as potatoes and corn.

The guidelines also called for substantial reductions in fat, saturated fat, and cholesterol. In addition to calling for less animal food consumption (2 to 3 servings a day), the report recommended that people "have cooked dry beans and peas instead of meat occasionally." Small amounts of dairy food (2 to 3 servings a day) were allowed, especially lowfat yogurt and skim milk. The report called for people to use sugars only in moderation.

Source: U.S. Department of Agriculture and U.S. Department of Health and Human Services, *Dietary Guidelines for Americans*, (Washington, D.C.: U.S. Government Printing Office, 1990).

29. The China Health Study

A Chinese research project, touted as the grand prix of epidemiology studies, challenged modern dietary assumptions in the early 1990s. Sponsored by the U.S. National Cancer Institute and the Chinese Institute of Nutrition and Food Hygiene, the study correlated average food and nutrient intakes with disease mortality rates in 65 rural Chinese counties. The typical Chinese diet included a high proportion of cereals and vegetables and a low content of meat, poultry, eggs, and milk. Less than 1 percent of deaths were caused by coronary heart disease, and breast cancer, colon cancer, lung cancer, and other malignancies common in the West were comparatively rare. Among the researchers' chief findings:

• Fat consumption should ideally be reduced to 10 to 15 percent of calories to prevent degenerative disease, not 30 percent as usually recommended.

• The lowest risk for cancer is generated by the consumption of a variety of fresh plant products.

• Eating animal protein is linked with chronic disease. Compared to the Chinese who derive 11 percent of their protein from animal sources, Americans obtain 70 percent from animal food.

• A rich diet that promotes early menstruation may increase a woman's risk of cancer of the breast and reproductive organs.

• Dairy food is not needed to prevent osteoporosis, the degenerative thinning of the bones that is common among older women.

• Meat consumption is not needed to prevent iron-deficiency anemia. The average Chinese consumes twice the iron Americans do, primarily from plant sources, and shows no signs of anemia.

Dr. T. Colin Campbell, a Cornell biochemist and principal American director of the project, noted, "Usually, the first thing a country does in the course of economic development is to introduce a lot of livestock. Our data are showing that this is not a very smart move, and the Chinese are listening. They're realizing that animal-

Comparison of Chinese and American Diets		
	China	U.S.
Dietary intakes		
Total dietary fibre (g/day)	33.3	11.1
Starch (g/day)	371	120
Plant protein (% of total protein)	89	30
Fat (% of calories)	14.5	38.8
Calcium (mg/day)	544	1143
Retinol (Vit. A retinol equiv/day)	27.8	990
Total carotenoids (retinol equiv/day)	836	429
Vitamic C (mg/day)	140	73
Blood plasma constituents		
Cholesterol (mg/dl	127	212
Triglycerides (mg/dl)	97	120
Total protein (g/dl)	4.8-6.2	6.4-8.3
Source: China Health Study, 1990		

based agriculture is not the way to go."

Source: Chen Junshi, T. Colin Campbell, Li Junyao, and Richard Peto, *Diet, Life-Style, and Mortality in China* (Ithaca, N.Y.: Cornell University Press, 1990). and Jane Brody, "Huge Study of Diet Indicts Fat and Meat," *New York Times*, May 8, 1990.

30. Physicians for Responsible Medicine

In 1991, the Physicians Committee for Responsible Medicine proposed four new food groups: whole grains; legumes (including beans and soy products such as tofu); vegetables; and fruits. This would replace the Four Basic Food Groups that have been the cornerstone of the modern way of eating: meat, fish and poultry; grains; dairy products; and fruits and vegetables. Meat, dairy, and other animal food would be minor options under the new proposed guidelines. "The typical Western diet, high in animal fat and protein and lacking in fiber, is associated with increased risk of cancer, heart disease, obesity, diabetes, and osteoporosis," a report issued by the 3,000-member doctors' group stated.

Source: "The New Four Food Groups," Physicians Committee for Responsible Medicine, Washington, D.C., April, 1991.

National and International Dietary Recommendations

	Limit Total Fat (% kcal)	Reduce Saturated Fat (% kcal)	Increase Polyunsat. Fat %kcal	Reduce Cholesterol mg/day	Limit Simple Sugars	Increase Complex Carbohydrates	Increase Fiber	Other Recommendations
General Health								
Standard Macrobiotic Diet (East West Foundation (1973)	~10-15	<2	Yes	Avoid	Avoid	~70-75	Yes	Organic grains and vegetables, miso, seaweed; chewing
Dietary Goals (1977)	27-33	10	to 10	300	Yes	55-60	Yes	Reduce additives, processed foods
Canada (1982)	35	Yes	Yes	No	Yes	Yes	Yes	Exercise
United Kingdom (1983)	30	10		No	20kg/yr	Yes	to 30 g/day	Exercise; nutrition education
Germany (1985)	Yes				Avoid excess	Yes	Yes	Variety; proper cooking
Japan Ministry of Health (1985)	20-25	Yes	Vegetable and fish oils					Variety; home cooking; pleasant environment
Sweden (1981, 1985)	25-35	Yes	Yes	Yes	<10%	50-60	>30 g/day	Variety; exercise; regular meals
Australia (1983, 1987)	33				<12%	Indirectly	30 g/day	Variety; promote breastfeeding
Diet and Health (1989)	≤30	≤10	7 to 10	<300	Yes	55	Yes	Limit protein; avoid supplements
China Health Study (1990)	~10	Yes	Yes	Yes	Yes	Yes	Yes	More plant foods; less animal food
Physicians for Responsible Medicine (1991)	15-20	Yes	Yes	Avoid	Avoid	70-75	Yes	Abolish 4 food groups; minimize animal food
Heart Disease								
American Heart Association (1988)	<30	<10	to 10	<300		50+		Variety of foods
World Health Organization (1982, 1990)	<20	<10	to 10	<300		Yes	>37	More plant foods, fish, low-fat
Multiple Heart Trial (Dr. Dean Ornish, 1990)	10	Yes	Yes	5	Yes	70-75	Yes	Avoid animal foods; eat soy products
Cancer								
National Academy of Sciences (1982)	~30	Yes	No		Yes			More whole grains, vegetables, fruits
American Cancer Society (1984)	~30	Yes	No			Yes	Yes	
Japan Panel on Nutrition (1983)	Avoid excess					Yes	Yes	Variety; chew well; seaweed

3

A Healthy Heart

Heart researchers have been in the forefront of dietary research since Russian scientists linked diet and atherosclerosis in the first decade of the century. In laboratory experiments in 1908, rabbits fed meat, milk, and eggs developed arterial lesions resembling atherosclerosis in humans, and cholesterol was subsequently identified as the principal dietary factor causing heart disease. After a half century of neglect, cardiovascular researchers begin to reexamine diet in the mid-1960s. In the early 1970s, the macrobiotic community in Boston became the focus of studies at Harvard Medical School and the Framingham Heart Study by Drs. Kass, Sacks, Castelli, and others. Along with Nathan Pritikin's pioneer work, these studies, showing that people eating little or no animal food and plenty of grains and vegetables had ideal blood pressure, cholesterol levels, and other heart values, revolutionized modern medicine's understanding of diet and heart disease. Since then, studies have been conducted showing that a balanced natural foods diet can not only prevent but also can reverse heart disease, the number one cause of death in modern society.

31. Korean War

Autopsies of young American men who died in the Korean war found evidence of widespread atheroslerosis. According to researchers, 77 percent of the men, whose average age was twenty-two, had grossly detectable coronary artery lesions, and 15 percent had coronary artery lesions that obstructed the arteries by 50 percent or more. Similar studies of young Korean casualties showed no evidence of atheroslerosis.

Source: W. F. Enos, R. H. Holmes, and J. Beyer, "Coronary Disease among United States Soldiers Killed in Action in Korea," *Journal of the American Medical Association* 152:1090-93, 1953.

32. Sea Vegetables, Shiitake, and Cholesterol

Japanese researchers reported that wakame, a common sea vegetable eaten in Asia, suppressed the reabsorption of cholesterol in the liver and intestine in laboratory experiments. Other studies showed that hijiki, another sea vegetable, and shiitake mushroom also lowered serum cholesterol and improved fat metabolism.

Source: N. Iritani and S. Nogi, "Effects of Spinach and Wakame on Cholesterol Turnover in the Rat," *Atherosclerosis* 15:87-92, 1972.

33. Harvard Macrobiotic Studies I

Harvard Medical School researchers reported a direct relation between blood pressure levels and articles of diet, especially the consumption of animal food. For four months, 210 men and women from many different backgrounds eating macrobiotically in Boston study houses were subjected to a wide range of medical tests. Overall, the researchers found that the men had mean systolic blood pressures of 109.7 mm Hg and diastolic pressures of 60.9. The women had slightly lower readings, 100.9 and 58.2 respectively. Both of these measurements fell well within the normal blood pressure category and approached the systolic level of 100 under which Framingham Heart Study researchers theorized there would develop virtually no coronary heart disease. Meanwhile, those in the group who ate fish or seafood regularly as a supplement to grains and vegetables had significantly higher blood pressure than those who ate no animal food. The addition of sea salt at the table was not associated with changes in blood pressure in those examined, and those individuals who abstained from coffee or cigarette smoking had lower systolic but not diastolic pressures. Married persons also had lower systolic pressures, as did those who meditated. The unexpectedly low blood pressure of the macrobiotic group was considered all the more remarkable because of the relatively short time the participants in the study had been on the new diet. "The generally short duration (less than 2 years) of adherence in half suggests that die-

Diet, Cholesterol, and Heart Disease

Population	Country	Diet	Average Cholesterol	Incidence of Heart Disease
Caucasian	U.S.A.	High-Fat, High-Sugar	220-280	High
Mediterranean	Greece, Italy, Yugoslavia	Low-Fat, Medium-Fiber	180-190	Moderate
Modern Rural	Japan, Latin America	Low-Fat, High-Fiber, Fish	150-160	Low
Inuit (Eskimo)	Canada	Fish & Vegetables	141	Low
Aborigines	Australia	Wild Plants & Animals	139	Rare
Rural Chinese	China	Grains & Vegetables	127	Rare
Macrobiotic	U.S.A.	Grains & Vegetables	126	Rare
Tarahumara	Mexico	Grains & Vegetables	125	Non-existent
Pygmies	Zaire	Wild Plants	110	Non-existent

Sources: New England Journal of Medicine, 1975, American Heart Association, 1980, American Journal of Medicine, 1986, China Health Study, 1990

tary effects on BP [blood pressure] become established relatively earlier. Perhaps of greater interest is that the declared intake of food from animal sources is significantly associated with higher pressures in individuals and there is signficant clustering of systolic BP among the members of communal households, a phenomenon hitherto observed only in relation to first-degree relatives of an individual and with varying degrees of association for spouses." The implications of these findings for a pluralistic society composed of many different racial and ethnic backgrounds were far-reaching.

Source: F. M. Sacks, Bernard Rosner, and Edward H. Kass, "Blood Pressure in Vegetarians," *American Journal of Epidemiology* 100:390-98, 1974.

34. Harvard Medical Studies II

Harvard Medical School researchers reported that Boston-area macrobiotic people eating a diet of whole grains, beans, fresh vegetables, sea vegetables, and fermented soy products had significantly lower cholesterol and triglyceride levels and lower blood pressure than a control group from the Framingham Heart Study eating the standard American diet of meat, sugar, dairy foods, and highly processed, chemicalized foods. The average serum cholesterol in the macrobiotic group was 126 milligrams per deciliter versus 184 for controls. When dairy foods and eggs were added to their diet, cholesterol and fat levels rose signficiantly, although fish was consumed as much as dairy and eggs combined. "The low plasma lipid levels in the vegetarians," the researchers concluded, "resemble those reported for populations in nonindustrialized societies" where heart disease, cancer, and other degenerative illnesses are uncommon.

Source:, F. M. Sacks et al., "Plasma Lipids and Lipoproteins in Vegetarians and Controls," *New England Journal of Medicine* 292:1148-51, 1975.

35. Harvard Medical Studies III

In one of the first studies to show the direct effects of animal food on raising blood pressure, a study of twenty-one macrobiotic persons by Harvard Medical School researchers found that the addition of 250 grams of beef per day for four weeks to their regular diet of whole grains and vegetables raised serum cholesterol levels 19 percent. Systolic blood pressure also rose significantly. After returning to a low-fat diet, cholesterol and blood pressure values returned to previous levels.

Source: F. M. Sacks et al., "Effects of Ingestion of Meat on Plasma Cholesterol of Vegetarians," *Journal of the American Medical Association* 246:640-44, 1981.

36. Diet and Blood Pressure

High blood pressure affects 15 to 20 percent of the adult population in the U.S. and other modern societies and is a leading cause of heart attack, stroke, and other cardiovascular diseases. For many years, modern medicine has assumed that blood pressure naturally rises with age. However, population studies in traditional societies have shown little or no tendency for blood pressure to increase with age. In a review of dietary changes among the Inuit, Polynesians, Bushmen, Central American Indians, and other native peoples, Lot B. Page, M.D. of the Tufts University School of Medicine found that in traditional societies abnormal blood pressure began to appear when people started eating the modern diet including refined salt, canned meat and fish, sugar, and other processed foods. In respect to salt, it was found that "acculturation, with use of Western dietary items, invariably appears to lead to increased salt intake." The researcher concluded that by eliminating these foods "clinical primary hypertension may be a preventable disease."

Source: Lot P. Page, "Epidemiologic Evidence on the Etiology of Human Hypertension and Its Possible Prevention," *American Heart Journal* 91:527-34, 1976.

37. Ni-Hon-San Study

Scientists observed that coronary heart disease prevalence and incidence rates tripled among Japanese within a generation of their migration to the West Coast of the United States and doubled in Japanese who migrated to Hawaii. These changes coincided with a change in the immigrants' diet, especially levels of saturated fat and serum cholestrol.

Source: T. L. Robertson et al., "Epidemiologic Studies of Coronary Heart Disease and Stroke in Japanese Men Living in Japan, Hawaii and California," *American Journal of Cardiology* 39:239-43, 1977.

38. Framingham Heart Study

Dr. William Castelli, director of the Framingham Heart Study, the nation's oldest and largest cardiovascular research project, and a participant in research on macrobiotic people at Harvard Medical School, noted that vegetarian and macrobiotic people have healthier hearts and circulatory systems than conditioned athletes:

"One of the most important issues of the 1980's is the question of reversibility of atherosclerosis. Most doctors have been taught that the process is irreversible; however, in most of the animal studies done, when animals with 90 percent of their blood vessels blocked by fatty deposits and scar tissue have had their cholesterol lowered to 150 mg. percent or lower, 80 percent of all lesions have disappeared in about four years. Case studies in humans have been documented in which blockages in the blood vessels have been reversed over time if the cholesterol level in the blood is lowered. In a study of 18,000 vegetarians in California it was found that they had only 15 percent of the heart attack rate reported in nonvegetarians. In addition, they have only 40 percent of the nonvegetarian cancer rate and the men live six to seven years longer than nonvegetarian men while vegetarian women live three years longer than non-vegetarian. . . .

"The study in Framingham suggests that the best way to determine how large the risk of heart attack is in a particular individual's life, is, to determine the ratio of his or her total cholesterol to HDL cholesterol. For example, a man with a total cholesterol of 200 and an HDL of 50 would have a ratio of 200/50 or 4. The majority of Americans who have heart attacks have a ratio of 4.6 to 5.7 so it is recommended that an individual's ratio be at least below 4.5. While getting one's ratio below 4.5 would not totally eliminate heart attack in this country, it would certainly change the fact that it is the number one killer in the U.S. now.

"What a person eats everyday is a very important aspect of how his or her health will be in everyday as well as later life. Supporting this view is the fact that macrobiotic people studied had a ratio of 2.5 and Boston marathon runners were at 3.4, ratios at which rarely, if ever, is coronary heart disease seen. Studies and observations such as these are a clear indicator that people need to take a critical look at their diet with the intention of making changes now."

Source: William P. Castelli, "Summary of Lessons from the Framingham Heart Study," Framingham, Mass., September, 1983.

39. The Oslo Study

In a study of 1,232 men aged 40 to 49 with high cholesterol who were put on a low-fat diet, reserchers found a 13 percent reduction in mean total cholesterol levels in comparison to a control group. At the end of 7.5 years, the incidence of heart attack and sudden death was 47 percent lower in the experimental group. The scientists attributed the changes to reduced cigarette smoking and diet.

Source: I. Hjermann, "Effect of Diet and Smoking Intervention on the Incidence of Coronary Heart Disease: Report from the Oslo Study Group of a Randomised Trial in Healthy Men," *Lancet* 2:1303-10, 1981.

40. Beans Lower Cholesterol

Men with high cholesterol who ate a diet including a half cup daily of dried pinto, navy, kidney, and other beans had an average drop in cholesterol levels of 20 percent after three weeks.

Source: J. W. Anderson and W. L. Chen, "Effects of Legumes and Their Soluble Fibers on Cholesterol-Rich Lipoproteins," *American Chemical Society Abstracts AGFD #39, 1982.*

41. Canadian Soyfoods Study

Scientists at the University of Western Ontario reported that the addition of soy protein in a person's diet could reduce serum cholesterol levels irrespective of other dietary considerations. In addition to animal studies, the researchers compared human volunteers who drank either cow's milk or soy milk and reported that "both cholesterol and triglyceride values dropped substantially during the soy period."

Source: *Journal of the American Medical Association* 247:3045-46, 1982.

42. Dutch Macrobiotic Study

Dutch heart researchers reported that macrobiotic men and boys had the most ideal cholesterol and other blood values in studies of groups of nonvegetarian, semi-lactovegetarian, lactovegetarian, and macrobiotic men aged thirty to thirty-nine years and boys aged six to eleven years old. The report was funded by the Netherlands Heart Foundation.

Source: J. T. Knuiman and C. E. West, "The Concentration of Cholesterol in Serum and in Various Serum Lipoproteins in Macrobiotic, Vegetarian, and Nonvegetarian Men and Boys," *Atherosclerosis* 43:71-82, 1983.

43. Belgian Macrobiotic Study

Researchers at the Academic Hospital of Ghent University in Belgium evaluated the blood values of twenty men assembled by Lima Natural Foods Factory who had an average age of thirty-six and had been macrobiotic for about eight years. According to the tests, all the men were very healthy. Their blood pressure and body weights were low, their hormone levels favorable, and they had normal vaues for proteins, vitamins, and minerals. Overall, their cholesterol values were significantly lower than ordinary people. J. P. Deslypere, M.D., one of the researchers, concluded, "[In] the field of cardiovascular and cancer risk factors this kind of blood is very favorable. It's ideal; we couldn't do better; that's what we're dreaming of. It's really fantastic, like children, whose blood vessels are still completely open and whole. This is a very important matter, deserving our full attention."

Source: Rik Vermuyten, *MacroMuse* (Fall/Metal 1984), p. 39.

44. Diet and Angina Pectoris

Physicians at Columbia Presbyterian Hospital in New York City reported that patients with angina pectoris, a form of coronary heart disease, showed significantly improved blood pressure values and lowered coronary risk factors after ten weeks on a macrobiotic diet and treatment with biofeedback in 1984. The chief researcher, Dr. Kenneth Greenspan of the hospital's Laboratory and Center for Stress Related Disorders, reported that cholesterol levels dropped from an average 300 to 220, levels of blood pressure also dropped, patients could walk about 20 percent farther in stress tests, and three patients with severe angina showed no symptoms at the end of the study. The participants, mostly businessmen, and their wives learned how to cook and ate together at the Natural Gourmet Cookery School under the direction of macrobiotic and natural foods cook Annemarie Colbin. Dr. Greenspan reported that there was "tremendous enthusiasm and adherence" to the new diet. The study was funded and monitored by the New York Cardiac Center.

Source: Michio Kushi and Alex Jack, *Diet for a Strong Heart* (New York: St. Martin's Press, 1985), p. 131.

45. Ireland-Boston Diet-Heart Study

Comparing the blood values of middle-aged Irishmen living in Ireland, their brothers who had migrated to Boston, and unrelated men of Irish descent living in Boston, researchers at Harvard School of Public Health found that mean total blood cholesterol levels were strongly correlated with intake of saturated fatty acid and dietary cholesterol from meat and other animal food. Fiber intake and vegetable consumption were also lower among those who died from coronary heart disease, leading the researchers to speculate that a decrease in complex carbohydrates rather than a change in fat consumption was the main causative factor in increased mortality from heart disease.

"Although the risk of coronary heart disease has been reported to be related to the intake of dietary lipids, an equally consistent finding has been the relation with starches and complex carbohydrates," the scientists noted. ". . . The principal nutritional change that has occurred since the early 1900s has been a decrease in the consumption of dietary carbohydrates, not including sugar, of about 45 percent during the period from 1909 to 1976. In contrast, changes in the consumption of dietary lipids have been much smaller."

Source: L. H. Kushi et al., "Diet and 20-Year Mortality from Coronary Heart Disease. The Ireland-Boston Diet-Heart Study," *New England Journal of Medicine* 312:811-18, 1985.

46. Ginger and Heart Disease

Ginger root can benefit the heart and circulatory system by slowing blood clotting. In studies at Mount Pleasant Hospital Addiction Studies Foundation in Lynn, Mass., ginger has been shown to inhibit thromboxane synthetase, a primary factor in platelet aggregation. Researchers noted that in contrast to drugs, ginger had minimal side-effects. "The indications for ginger as a therapeutic agent may be far reaching in psychiatry and medicine," the scientists concluded.

Source: J. Backon, "Inhibition of Thromboxane Synthetase and Stimulation of Prostacylin: Relevance for Medicine and Psychiatry," *Medical Hypotheses* 20:271, 1986.

47. Dr. Dean Ornish's Lifestyle Heart Trial

Dietary and lifestyle changes alone can prevent or reverse hardening of the arteries. In the first random case-control clinical trial to determine whether patients outside the hospital can be motivated to make and sustain comprensive lifestyle changes, 82 percent of patients with heart disease who were put on a low-fat, vegetarian diet, who exercised, and who were given stress-management training including yoga and meditation had a measurable widening of arteries. In contrast, those who observed the moderate American Heart Association diet and received customary care such as drugs and surgery had an increase in blockages.

The experimental diet consisted primarily of whole grains, beans, legumes, and soybean products (including tofu), vegetables, fruits, and no animal food except for small amounts of egg white

Diet and Reversal of Coronary Heart Disease		
	Vegetarian Diet	**Standard Diet***
Total Cholesterol	Down 24.3%	Down 5.4%
LDL Cholesterol	Down 37.4%	Down 5.8%
Blood Pressure	127/79	131/77
Angina Frequency	Down 91%	Up 165%
Angina Duration	Down 42%	Up 95%
Angina Severity	Down 28%	Up 39%
Clogging of Arteries	Down 2.2%	Up 3.4%
Severe Clogging	Down 5.3%	Up 2.7%
Atherosclerotic Progress	18 of 22 Subjects Improved	10 of 19 Subjects Worsened

* Controls were given the American Heart Association Diet (with fat allowed to 30% kcal) which was considered "prudent."

Source: *Lancet, 1990*

and nonfat milk or yogurt. The stress management techniques included stretching exercises, breathing techniques, meditation, progressive relaxation, and imagery.

Before treatment, doctors found that coronary arteries in the patients were blocked an average of 40 percent. After one year on a diet with only 10 percent fat, the average blockage improved to 37.8 percent. According to principal researcher Dean Ornish of the Preventive Medicine Research Institute in Sausalito, California, the greatest improvement was in the arteries that had been the most clogged. In contrast, the coronary blockages in the control group who received conventional treatment increased from 42.7 percent to 46.1 percent.

Eighteen of twenty-two patients in the experiment group experienced healing in damaged arteries, while ten of nineteen patients in the control group worsened. Cholesterol in the low-fat group dropped from an average of 213 to 154 a year later. Those on the special diet also reported a 91 percent drop in the frequency of angina, while those in the control group reported a 165 percent rise in angina.

"This clinical trial has show that a heterogeneous group of patients with coronary heart disease can be motivated to make comprehensive changes in lifestyle for at least a year outside hospital," researchers concluded. "This finding suggests that conventional recommendations for patients with coronary heart disease (such as a 30 percent fat diet) are not sufficient to bring about regression in many patients."

In his popular program to prevent and relieve heart disease, Dr. Ornish recommends many macrobiotic quality foods including brown rice, miso soup, tempeh, tofu, and amazake.

Sources: Dean Ornish et al., "Can Lifestyle Changes Reverse Coronary Heart Disease?" *Lancet* 336:129-33, 1990 and Dean Ornish, *Dr. Dean Ornish's Program for Reversing Heart Disease* (New York: Random House, 1990).

48. Heart Disease Trends

Coronary heart disease deaths declined 46.3 percent in the United States since 1968, largely as a result of changing food consumption, according to scientists who reviewed 171 studies published since 1920.

U.S. average per capita fat consumption increased from 34 percent of calories in the 1930s to 40 to 44 percent in the late 1950s for men and 40 to 44 percent in the mid-1960s for women and children. Since the 1960s, fat consumption has steadily fallen to about 36 percent in 1984.

The type of fat ingested has also changed. In the early 1950s, saturated and monounsaturated fat accounted for 18 to 20 percent of calories, while in the mid-1980s it fell to 12 to 13 percent. Over the same period, polyunsaturated fats increased from between 2 and 4 percent to 7.5 percent.

Source: Alison M. Stephen and Nicholas J. Wald, "Trends in Individual Consumption of Dietary Fat in the United States, 1920-1984," *American Journal of Clinical Nutrition* 52:457-69, 1990.

49. Multiple Risk Factor Intervention Trial

A study of more than 12,000 men of middle age found that reducing cholesterol by 5 percent, lowering blood pressure, losing weight, and receiving help to stop smoking substantially reduced the risk of heart attack. The research followed the men over a period of ten years and found that the half which made dietary and lifestyle changes had 24 percent fewer deaths from heart attack than the control group which received conventional medical care.

Source: "Mortality Rates after 10.5 Years for Participants in the Multiple Risk Factor Intervention Trial," *Journal of the American Medical Association* 263:1795-1801, 1990.

50. Vegetables and Heart Disease

Vegetables and fruits high in beta-carotene can reduce the risk of heart disease by about half in people with clogged coronary arteries. In a report to the American Heart Association, researchers followed 333 male doctors who had coronary artery disease. After six years of study, the men who took beta carotene supplements had ten heart attacks compared to seventeen in the placebo group.

Beta carotene is found primarily in orange and yellow vegetables such as carrots and squash and in yellow fruits such as apricots, peaches, and cantaloupes. Kale and other green leafy vegetables also are high in beta-carotene.

Source: "Type of Vitamin A May Reduce Heart Ills," *Boston Globe*, November 14, 1990.

51. Rice Bran Oil

Rice bran oil protects against heart disease, according to research presented to the American Heart Association. In studies with monkeys, rice bran oil lowered harmful LDL cholesterol by up to 30 percent without reducing beneficial HDL cholesterol that helps prevent heart attacks. Rice bran oil was also found to contain substances that impede the deposit of cholesterol inside arteries.

Source: "Oil from Rice Aids Monkey," *New York Times*, January 15, 1991.

4
Cancer Prevention

Despite many epidemiological studies, animal studies, and personal accounts from cancer patients, the scientific and medical community was relatively slow to recognize the link between diet and cancer. The National Academy of Sciences' 1982 study, Diet, Nutrition, and Cancer, is the most comprehensive survey to date of this relationship. In the last decade, all of the major medical associations issued dietary guidelines in the direction of a more balanced diet. As in the case of heart disease, current research is showing that whole grains, vegetables, and other whole natural foods are remedial as well as preventive. Miso, tofu, kombu, shiitake mushroom, and other foods have been shown to be particularly beneficial.

52. Cancer and Longevity in Japan

Epidemiologists reported that cancer of the lung, breast, and colon increased two to three times among Japanese women between 1950 and 1975. During that period, milk consumption increased fifteen times; meat, eggs, and poultry climbed seven and a half times; and rice consumption dropped 70 percent. In Okinawa, with the highest proportion of centenarians, longevity was associated with lowered sugar and salt intake and higher intake of protein and green and yellow vegetables.

Source: Y. Kagawa, "Impact of Westernization on the Nutrition of Japan," *Preventive Medicine* 7:205-17, 1978.

53. Diet vs. Conventional Treatment

In 1985 the National Cancer Institute reported that radiation therapy and chemotherapy were ineffective and in some cases produced toxic side-effects as follow-ups to surgery in the treatment of cancer. "Except possibly in selected patients with cancer of the stomach, there has been no demonstrated improvement in the survival of patients with the ten most common cancers when radiation therapy, chemotherapy, or both have been added to surgical resection." The ten most common cancers include lung, colorectum, breast, prostate, uterus, bladder, pancreas, stomach, skin, and kidney. Shortly after the report was published, the author, Dr. Steven A. Rosenberg, the N.C.I.'s chief of surgery, operated on President Ronald Reagan's colon cancer and instead of chemotherapy or radiation treatment put him on a modified whole grain diet.

Source: Steven A. Rosenberg, "Combined-Modality Therapy of Cancer," *New England Journal of Medicine* 312:1512-14 and Alex Jack, personal communication with the White House, July, 1985.

54. Soybeans and Breast Cancer

Scientists reported that a diet high in soybeans reduced the incidence of breast cancer in laboratory experiments. The active ingredient in the soybeans was identified as protease inhibitors, also found in certain other beans and seeds.

Source: W. Troll, "Blocking of Tumor Promotion by Protease Inhibitors," in J. H. Burchenal and H. F. Oettgen (eds.), *Cancer: Achievements, Challenges, and Prospects for the 1980s, Vol. 1*, New York: Grune and Stratton, pp. 549-55, 1980.

55. Macrobiotics and Breast Cancer

Macrobiotic and vegetarian women are less likely to develop breast cancer, researchers at New England Medical Center in Boston reported. The scientists found that macrobiotic and vegetarian women process estrogen differently from other women and eliminate it more quickly from their body. The study involved forty-five pre- and postmenopausal women, about half of whom were macrobiotic and vegetarian and half nonvegetarian. The women consumed about the same number of total calories. Although the vegetarian women took in only one third as much animal protein and animal fat, they excreted two to three times as much estrogen. High levels of estrogen have been associated with the development of breast cancer. "The difference in estrogen metabolism may explain the lower incidence of breast cancer in vegetarian women," the study concluded.

Source: B. R. Goldin et al., "Effect of Diet on Excretion of Estrogens in Pre- and Postmenopausal Incidence of Breast Cancer in Vegetarian Women," *Cancer Research* 41:3771-73, 1981.

Correlations Between Female Cancers and Dietary Variables					
Variables*	Breast		Uterine	Ovary	
	Incidence	Mortality	Incidence	Incidence	Mortality
Cereals	-0.64	-0.70	-0.58	-0.43	-0.78
Pulses	-0.43	-0.46	-0.62	-0.41	-0.53
Fruits	0.64	0.44	0.54	0.16	0.31
Meat	0.78	0.74	0.78	0.40	0.53
Eggs	0.71	0.80	0.68	0.28	0.51
Milk	0.66	0.73	0.64	0.47	0.66
Sugar	0.70	0.74	0.62	0.43	0.78
Coffee	0.42	0.37	0.43	0.50	0.50

* Negative numbers such as all cereal and pulse measures show an inverse correlation or a protective value.

Source: International Journal of Cancer, 1975

56. Sea Vegetables and Breast Cancer

In an experiment at the Harvard School of Public Health, laboratory animals fed a control diet with 5 percent *Laminaria* (kombu), a brown sea vegetable, developed induced mammary cancer later than animals not fed seaweed. "Seaweed has shown consistent antitumor activity in several *in vivo* animal tests," the researcher concluded. "In extrapolating these results to the Japanese population, seaweed may be an important factor in explaining the low rates of certain cancers in Japan. Breast cancer shows a three-fold-lower rate among premenopausal Japanese women and a nine-fold-lower rate among postmenopausal women in Japan than reported for women in the United States. Since low levels of exposure to some toxic substances have been shown to be carcinogenic, then it may be that low levels of daily intake of food with antitumor properties may reduce cancer incidence."

Source: J. Teas, M. L. Harbison, and R. S. Gelman, "Dietary Seaweed [*Laminaria*] and Mammary Carcinogenesis in Rats," *Cancer Research* 44:2758-61, 1984.

57. Sea Vegetables and Breast Cancer

In Japan, tests on six groups of female rats showed that adding sea vegetables to the diet resulted in significant inhibitory effect on induced mammary tumorigenesis. "Tumor incidences were 35 percent (7/20), 35 percent (7/20) and 50 percent (9/18), respectively [for groups fed nori, kombu, and another type of kombu], whereas that in the control group was 69 percent (920/29)," investigators reported. The onset of tumors was also delayed in the seaweed groups, and the weight of tumors was lower.

Source: Ichiro Yamamoto et al., "The Effect of Dietary Seaweeds on 7,12-Dimethyl-Benz[a]Anthracene-Induced Mammary Tumorigenesis in Rats," *Cancer Letters* 35:109-18, 1987.

58. Dairy and Breast Cancer

Dairy food may be the most potent factor in the development of breast cancer. A study of 250 women with breast cancer in the northwestern province of Vercelli, Italy, found that they tended to consume considerably more milk, high-fat cheese, and butter than 499 healthy women of the same age in Italy and France.

Breast cancer risk tripled among women who consumed about half their calories as fat, 13 to 23 percent of their calories as saturated fat, and 8 to 20 percent of their calories as animal protein.

"These data suggest that during adult life, a reduction in dietary intake of fat and proteins of animal origin may contribute to a substantial reduction in the incidence of breast cancer in population subgroups with high intake of animal products," researchers concluded. "[A] diet rich in fat, saturated fat, or animal proteins may be associated with a twofold to threefold increase in a woman's risk of breast cancer."

Source: Paolo Toniolo et al., "Calorie-Providing Nutrients and Risk of Breast Cancer," *Journal of the National Cancer Institute* 81:278-86, 1989.

59. Miso and Breast Cancer

The incidence of breast cancer in first-generation Japanese migrants to Hawaii is about 60 percent of the rate in subsequent generations of Japanese born in Hawaii. Researchers at the Departments of Nutrition Sciences and Biostatistics/Biomathematics, University of Alabama at Birmingham, theorized that miso, natto, tamari soy sauce, and other traditionally fermented soybean foods may contribute to lowered disease. The consumption of these foods in Japan is about five times or more what it is among Japanese migrants to Hawaii.

To test their hypothesis, the scientists initiated feeding trials with rats and found that feeding miso to the rats delayed the appearance of induced breast cancer compared with animals on the control diet. The miso- and salt-supplemented diet treatment group showed a trend toward a lower number of cancers per animal, a trend toward a higher number of benign tumors per animal, and a trend toward a lower growth rate of cancers compared with controls.

"This data suggest that miso consumption may be a factor producing a lower breast cancer incidence in Japanese women," the researchers concluded. "Organic compounds found in fermented soybean-based foods may exert a chemoprotective effect."

Source: J. E. Baggott et al., "Effect of Miso (Japanese Soybean Paste) and NaCl on DMBA-Induced Rat Mammary Tumors," *Nutrition and Cancer* 14:103-09, 1990.

60. Fiber and Breast Cancer

Whole grains, cereals, and other foods high in fiber may help protect against breast cancer. In laboratory tests, scientists at the American Health Foundation found that a high-fiber diet reduced induced cancer in rats by about 50 percent. "We found that by doubling the amount of fiber in a diet that is similar to our Western diet, you can significantly reduce the amount of mammary cancer," concluded researcher Leonard Cohen.

Sources: L. A. Cohen et al., "Modulation of N-Nitrosomethylurea-Induced Mammary Tumor Promotion by Dietary Fiber and Fat," *Journal of the National Cancer Institute*, 83:496-500, 1991 and "Fiber Is Linked to Reduced Breast Cancer Risk," *Boston Globe*, April 3, 1991.

61. Japanese Migrants

In 1968 an epidemiological study indicated that dietary habits and environmental influences are the chief determinants of the world's varying cancer rates and not genetic factors. Data showed that in the course of three generations, Japanese migrants in the United States contracted colon cancer at the same rates as the general American population. In contrast, the regular colon cancer rate in Japan remained about one-fourth the American incidence.

Source: W. Haenszel and M. Kurihara, "Studies of Japanese Migrants," *Journal of the National Cancer Institute* 40:43-68.

62. Diet and Colon Cancer

• Men in Finland consume a lot of fat and have the highest heart disease rate in the industrialized world. Yet they have one of the lowest colon cancer rates (one-third that of the U.S.). Researchers around the world have found that whole cereal grains protect against colon cancer by reducing bile acid concentrates in the large intestine and giving bulk to the feces. Investigators found that Finnish men consume high amounts of whole rye bread and had bowel movements three times bulkier than men in other Western countries as well as reduced amounts of bile acid buildup.

Source: H. N. Englyst et al., "Nonstarch Polysaccharide Concentrations in Four Scandinavian Populations,"*Nutrition & Cancer* 4:50-60, 1982.

• Eating more whole grains, vegetables, and fruit may lower a person's risk for colorectal cancer by up to 40 percent. Researchers at the Fox Chase Cancer Center in Philadelphia looked at thirty-seven studies involving 10,000 people in fifteen countries and reported that those who ate a diet high in whole grains and other plant-quality foods had about 40 percent less risk of this disease.

Source: Bruce Tock, Elaine Lanza, and Peter Greenwald, "Dietary Fiber, Vegetables, and Colon Cancer: Critical Review and Meta-analyses of the Epidemiologic Evidence," *Journal of the National Cancer Institute* 82:650-661, 1990.

• Researchers at Harvard School of Public Health reported that men with the lowest fat intake, averaging 24 percent of calories, had only half the rate of colon polyps, a common precursor of colon cancer, as men eating the usual amount of fat. "A modest reduction [of fat such as proposed by current medical guidelines] will not appreciably reduce the risk," said Dr. Tim Byers of the Center for Disease Control in Atlanta. He described an effective cancer-prevention diet as one that included six servings a day of whole grains and legumes and five or six servings of vegetables and fruits.

Source: "Very Low Rate of Fat in Diet Is Advised to Fight Cancer," *Boston Globe*, April 23, 1991.

63. Cruciferous Vegetables and Colon Cancer

In Norway, researchers examined the colons of 155 people in their fifties who had no signs of colon cancer. Half had polyps growing in the colon; the half with no polyps ate more cruciferous vegetables. The less cruciferous vegetables consumed, the greater the risk for polyps and the larger and more abnormal the polyps.

Source: G. Hoff et. al., *Scandinavian Journal of Gastroenterology* 21:199, 1986.

64. Beans and Bile Acids

Beans lowered bile acid production by 30 percent in men with a tendency toward elevated bile acid. Bile acids are necessary for proper fat digestion but in excess have been associated with causing cancer, especially in the large intestine. Case-control studies showed that pinto and navy beans were effective in lowering bile acid production in men at high risk for this condition.

Source: J. W. Anderson, "Hypocholesterolemic Effects of Oat-Bran or Bean Intake for Hypercholesterolemic Men," *American Journal of Clinical Nutrition* 40:1146-55, 1984.

65. Nurses' Health Study and Colon Cancer

Women who eat beef, lamb, or pork as a daily main dish are at two and a half times the risk for developing colon cancer as women who eat meat less than once a month. The conclusion, drawn from a study of 88,751 nurses, over a ten-year period, found that the more fish and poultry in the diet the less chances of getting colon cancer. "The substitution of other protein sources, such as beans or lentils, for red meat might also be associated with a reduced risk of colon cancer in populations that consume more legumes," researchers concluded. Investigators also found that eating the fiber from fruit appeared to reduce the risk of colon cancer. The fruits mentioned as possibly protective included apples and pears.

"The less red meat the better," recommended Dr. Walter Willett, professor of epidemiology and nutrition at the Harvard School of Public Health, who directed the study. "At most, it should be eaten only occasionally. And it may be maximally effective not to eat red meat at all."

Sources: Walter C. Willett et al., "Relation of Meat, Fat, and Fiber Intake to the Risk of Colon Cancer in a Prospective Study among Women," *New England Journal of Medicine* 323:1664-72, 1990 and Anastasia Toufexis, "Red Alert on Red Meat," *Time,* December 24, 1990.

66. Lentils and Esophageal Tumors

A study in the Caspian littoral region of Iran, an area of high esophageal cancer, associated this disease with lower intake of lentils and other pulses, cooked green vegetables, and other whole foods.

Source: H. Hormozdiari et al., "Dietary Factors and Esophageal Cancer in the Caspian Littoral of Iran," *Cancer Research* 35:3493-98, 1975.

67. Fiber and Esophageal Cancer

An epidemiological study found that populations with a low risk of esophageal cancer in Africa and Asia consume more millet, cassava, yams, peanuts, and other foods high in fiber or starch than high-risk groups.

Source: S. J. van Rensburg, "Epidemiologic and Dietary Evidence for a Specific Nutritional Predisposition to Esophageal Cancer," *Journal of the National Cancer Institute* 67:243-51, 1981.

68. Diet and Leukemia

In 1972 a Japanese scientist reported that leukemia in chickens could be reversed by feeding them a mixture of whole grains and salt. The experiment was conducted by Keiichi Morishita, M.D., technical chief for the Tokyo Red Cross Blood Center and vice president of the New Blood Association.

Source: K. Morishita, M.D., *The Hidden Truth of Cancer* (San Francisco: George Ohsawa Macrobiotic Foundation, 1972).

69. Vegetables and Lung Cancer

A Chicago study found that regular consumption of foods containing beta carotene, a precursor to vitamin A, protected against lung cancer. Over a period of nineteen years, a group of 1,954 men at a Western Electric plant were monitored, and those who regularly consumed carrots, dark green lettuce, spinach, broccoli, kale, Chinese cabbage, peaches, apricots, and other carotene-rich foods had significantly lower lung cancer rates than controls.

Source: R. B. Shekelle et al., "Dietary Vitamin A and Risk of Cancer in the Western Electric Study," *Lancet* 2:1185-90, 1981.

70. Fat and Lung Cancer

In a review of the relation of diet, lifestyle, and lung cancer, researchers found that calories from dietary fat were highly significantly associated with lung cancer mortality. For example, male lung cancer deaths are highest in West European countries where a high-fat diet is consumed, and lowest in Thailand, Philippines, Honduras, Guatemala, and Japan where a low-fat diet is eaten.

While noting that smoking is still the major causative factor of lung cancer, the scientists theorized that a high-fat diet might also trigger the process by which cigarette smoke is harmful to the lungs. It is conceivable that "tobacco smoke is readily oxidized to the ultimate carcinogen as a consequence of a high-fat diet."

Source: Ernst L. Wynder, James R. Hebert, and Geoffrey Kabat, "Association of Dietary Fat and Lung Cancer," *Journal of the National Cancer Institute* 79:631-37, 1987.

71. Lymphoma and Diet

Persons who regularly eat cereal grains, pulses, vegetables, seeds, and nuts are less likely to get lymphoma or Hodgkin's disease than persons who do not usually eat these foods, according to a 1976 survey based on World Health Organization data.

Source: A. S. Cunningham, "Lymphomas and Animal-Protein Consumption," *Lancet* 2:1184-86.

72. Dairy and Ovarian Cancer

Dairy food consumption has been linked with ovarian cancer

by researchers at Harvard. The scientists noted that women with ovarian cancer had low blood levels of transferase, an enzyme involved in the metabolism of dairy foods. The researchers theorized that women with low levels of transferase who eat dairy foods, especially yogurt and cottage cheese, could increase their risk of ovarian cancer by as much as three times.

The researchers estimated that women who consume large amounts of yogurt and cottage cheese increased their risk of ovarian cancer up to three times.

"Yogurt was consumed at least monthly by 49 percent of cases and 36 percent of controls," researchers reported. "World wide, ovarian cancer risk is strongly correlated with lactase persistence and per capita milk consumption, further epidemiological evidence that lactose rather than fat is the key dietary variable for ovarian cancer . . . [A]voidance of lactose-rich food by adults may be a way of primary prevention of ovarian cancer . . . "

Source: Daniel W. Cramer et al., "Galactose Consumption and Metabolism in Relation to the Risk of Ovarian Cancer," *Lancet* 2:66-71, 1989.

73. Shiitake and Sarcomas

Japanese scientists at the National Cancer Center Research Institute reported that shiitake mushrooms had a strong anti-tumor effect. In experiments with mice, polysaccharide preparations from various natural sources, including the shiitake mushroom commonly available in Tokyo markets, markedly inhibited the growth of induced sarcomas resulting in "almost complete regression of tumors . . . with no sign of toxicity."

Source: G. Chihara et al., "Fractionation and Purification of the Polysaccharides with Marked Antitumor Activity, Especially Lentinan, from *Lentinus edodes* (Berk.) Sing. (An Edible Mushroom)," *Cancer Research* 30:2776-81, 1970.

74. Sea Vegetables and Sarcomas

Japanese scientists reported that several varieties of kombu and mojaban, common sea vegetables eaten in Asia and traditionally used as a decoction for cancer in Chinese herbal medicine, were effective in the treatment of tumors in laboratory experiments. In three of four samples tested, inhibition rates in mice with implanted sarcomas ranged from 89 to 95 percent. The researchers reported

Antitumor Effect of Seaweeds on Sarcomas in Mice					
Sample	Dose (mg/kg)	Average tumor weight (g.)	Inhibition ratio	Complete regression	Mortality
Sargassum fulvellum	100 x 10	0.18	89.3%	7/9	1/10
Control		1.67		0/10	0/10
Laminaria angustata	100 x 5	0.08	94.8%	6/9	1/10
Control		1.59		0/10	0/10
Laminaria angustata var. longissima	100 x 5	0.21	92.3%	5/9	1/10
Control		2.71		0/7	0/7
Laminaria japonica	100 x 5	1.40	13.6%	2/9	1/10
Control		1.62		0/9	1/10
Source: *Japanese Journal of Experimental Medicine, 1974*					

that "the tumor underwent complete regression in more than half of the mice of each treated group." Similar experiments on mice with leukemia showed promising results.

Source: I. Yamamoto et al., "Antitumor Effect of Seaweeds," *Japanese Journal of Experimental Medicine* 44:543-46, 1974.

75. Tofu and Stomach Cancer

Japanese cancer researchers found that people who regularly ate tofu were at less risk for stomach cancer than those who did not.

Source: T. Hirayama, "Epidemiology of Stomach Cancer," in T. Murakami (ed.), *Early Gastric Cancer. Gann Monograph on Cancer Research,* 11 (Tokyo: University of Tokyo Press, pp. 3-19), 1971.

Relation of Miso Intake, Cancer, and Disease				
	Miso Soup Consumption			
Cause of Death*	Daily	Occasionally	Rarely	Never
Stomach Cancer	Baseline	Up 18%	Up 34%	Up 48%
Cancer at All Sites	Baseline	Up 4%	Up 12%	Up 19%
Coronary Heart Disease	Baseline	Up 7%	Up 10%	Up 43%
High Blood Pressure	Baseline	Up 29%	Up 11%	Up 453%
Cerebrovascular Disease	Baseline	Down 11%	Down 13%	Up 29%
Liver Cirrhosis	Baseline	Up 25%	Up 25%	Up 57%
Peptic Ulcer	Baseline	Up 17%	Up 41%	Up 52%
All Causes of Death	Baseline	Up 2%	Up 6%	Up 33%

*Association of age-sex standardized rate ratio for major causes of death, 1966-78.
Source: *Nutrition and Cancer, 1982*

76. Miso Soup and Stomach Cancer

Japan's National Cancer Center reported that people who eat miso soup daily are 33 percent less likely to contract stomach cancer and 19 percent less likely to contract cancer at other sites than those who never eat miso soup. The thirteen-year study, involving about 265,000 men and women over forty, also found that those who never ate miso soup had a 43 percent higher death rate from coronary heart disease than those who consumed miso soup daily. Those who abstained from miso also had 29 percent more fatal strokes, three and a half times more deaths resulting from high blood pressure, and higher mortality from all other causes.

Source: T. Hirayama, "Relationship of Soybean Paste Soup Intake to Gastric Cancer Risk," *Nutrition and Cancer* 3:223-33, 1981.

77. Macrobiotic Case Histories

Over the last several decades there have been scores of case history reports published by or about individuals with cancer who have benefited from a macrobiotic dietary approach. The major cancer recovery cases published in book form with varying degrees of medical documentation include:

• Jean Kohler, a music professor at Ball State University in Indiania, who had terminal pancreatic cancer.

• Virginia Brown, R.N., a nurse from Vermont who had malignant melanoma, Stage IV.

• Elaine Nussbaum, a New Jersey housewife with an inoperable uterine tumor.

• Kit Kitatani, a United Nations administrator from Japan, who had untreatable stomach cancer.

• Norman Arnold, a Southern businessman with pancreatic cancer.

• Hugh Faulkner, M.D., a British doctor with pancreatic cancer.

• Christina Pirello, who had untreatable leukemia.

Sources: Jean and Mary Alice Kohler, *Healing Miracles from Macrobiotics* (West Nyack, N.Y.: Parker, 1979); Virginia Brown with Susan Stayman, *Macrobiotic Miracle: How A Vermont Family Overcame Cancer* (Tokyo and New York: Japan Publications, 1984); Elaine Nussbaum, *Recovery: From Cancer to Health Through Macrobiotics* (Tokyo and New York: Japan Publications, 1986); Kit Kitatani, Norman Arnold, Hugh Faulker, and Christina Pirello in Ann Fawcett and the East West Foundation, *Cancer-Free:* (Tokyo and New York: Japan Publications, 1991).

78. Research on Cancer and Macrobiotics

• In a study of twenty-four patients with pancreatic cancer who adopted a macrobiotic diet, Tulane University researchers found that their mean length of survival was 17.3 months, compared with 6.0 months for matched controls from a national tumor registry diagnosed during the same time period (1984-85). The one-year survival rate was 54.2 percent in the macrobiotic patients versus 10.0 percent in the controls. All comparisons were statistically significant.

Source: Gordon Saxe, "A Retrospective Study of Diet and Cancer of the Pancreas," in Ann Fawcett, *Cancer-Free* (Tokyo and New York: Japan Publications, 1991).

• In a study of patients with advanced malignancies who followed a macrobiotic way of eating, Vivien Newbold, M.D., a Philadelphia physician documented six cases of remission. The patients had pancreatic cancer with metastases to the liver; malignant melanoma; malignant astrocytoma; endometrial stromal sarcoma; adenocarcinoma of the colon; and inoperable intra-abdominal leimyosarcoma. Review of CT scans and other medical tests revealed no evidence of tumors after adherence to the macrobiotic diet. All of the patients (except for one whose cancer came back after she discontinued macrobiotics) were reported working full time, leading very active lives, and feeling in excellent health. The cases were all reviewed independently and the diagnoses confirmed by the pathology and radiology departments of Holy Redeemer Hospital in Meadowbrook, Pa. In a review of her study, Congressional investigators recommended further research on the macrobiotic approach to cancer: "If cases such as Newbold's were presented in the medical literature, it might help stimulate interest among clinical investigators in conducting controlled, prospective trials of macrobiotic regimens, which could provide valid data on effectiveness."

Source: Office of Technology Assessment (OTA), *Unconventional Cancer Treatments* (Washington, D.C.: Government Printing Office, 1990).

79. Chewing and Cancer

An Indian cancer researcher concluded that thorough chewing lowered the risk of cancer. "The proper chewing of meals ensuring that mucous-rich saliva mixed with the food seemed to be protective factors." Cancer also appeared to more prevalent in south India where white rice and considerably more fat, oil, and spices are used in cooking than in north India where whole-grain chapatis and thick dal made with lentils are the staple.

Source: S. L. Malhotra, "Dietary Factors in a Study of Cancer Colon from Cancer Registry, with Special Reference to the Role of Saliva, Milk and Fermented Milk Products, and Vegetable Fibre," *Medical Hypotheses* 3:122-26, 1977.

80. Soy Sauce and Cancer

The high rate of stomach cancer in Japan caused some Japanese scientists to speculate that a diet high in soy sauce might be a factor. However, researchers at the University of Wisconsin observed just the opposite. In laboratory tests, mice given fermented soy sauce experienced 26 percent less cancer than mice on the regular diet. Also soy-supplemented mice averaged about one-quarter the number of tumors per mouse as the control group. Soy sauce "exhibited a pronounced anticarcinogenic effect," the researchers concluded.

Source: J. Raloff, "A Soy Sauce Surprise," *Science News*, 139:357, 1991.

5

Avoiding Common Disorders A to Z

Though most nutritional research has focused on heart disease and cancer, the two most life-threatening diseases, many other chronic illnesses have also been linked with immoderate food intake. Dietary changes have also proved effective in preventing or relieving a variety of common conditions and in emergency first-aid.

81. Acne

A doctor reported that patients who took one ounce of high-fiber breakfast cereal every day showed rapid clearing up of acne. He speculated that "a diet low in fat, salt, and refined carbohydrates and high in vegetable fibre" could be of value in the management of acne by reducing constipation which has been associated with this skin affliction.

Source: W. F. Kaufman, "The Diet and Acne," [Letter], *Archives of Dermatology* 119:276, 1983.

82. Allergies

In food trials, a teenage boy in the hospital with muscular and skeletal pains, bronchial asthma, abdominal pains, headache, and dark circles under the eyes experienced substantial improvement within two days when milk and chocolate were taken out of the diet. "Within forty-eight hours the facial pallor and the dark circles under his eyes almost completely disappeared. Most remarkable was the improvement in his mood and behavior. He became alert and interested in his surroundings, was surprisingly cheerful and began to take a keen interest in sporting activities and art classes at which he excelled. He no longer complained of vague aches and pains. His asthma was easily controlled." Following three weeks of the therapeutic diet, milk was given to him again and the pallor, dark circles, and other symptoms returned.

Source: E. G. Weinberg and M. Tuchinda, "Allergic Tension-Fatigue Syndrome," *Annals of Allergy* 31:209-11, 1973.

83. Alzheimer's Disease

About 1.5 to 2 million Americans have Alzheimer's disease, and it is now the fourth leading cause of death in the nation. While the exact cause of this condition that is characterized by progressive loss of memory and intellectual abilities has not been identified, research has discovered high amounts of aluminum concentrates in the plaque and neurofibrillary tangles in the brains of Alzheimer patients. Some scientists speculate that this is caused by aluminum additives in food and drugs, the use of aluminum foil and cookware, and toxins in the water supply.

• In England doctors reported that water prepared in aluminum coffee pots showed thirty times as much aluminum as the acceptabled level recommended by the World Health Organization. Boiling the water caused the levels of aluminum to rise from 22 mcg. to 1,640 mcg. in a liter of water. Another team of British researchers found a causal connection between aluminum concentrations in drinking water in eighty-eight counties in England and Wales over a 10-year period and reported incidence of Alzheimer's disease.

Sources: James A. Jackson, Hugh Riordan, and C. Milton Poling, "Aluminum from a Coffee Pot," [Letter], *Lancet* 1:781, 1989; C.N. Martyn et al., "Geographical Relation Between Alzheimer's Disease and Aluminium in Drinking Water," *Lancet*, January 14, 1989, pp. 59-62.

• Studies have found that people with Alzheimer's disease have reduced levels of acetylcholine, a neurotransmitter, in the brain that is stimulated by dietary factors such as choline and lecithin, a substance found naturally in soybeans and other legumes.

Source: R. J. Wurtman, "Alzheimer's Disease," *Scientific-American* 252:62-74, 1985.

84. Arthritis

• Twelve of twenty patients aged thirty-five to sixty-eight put on a strict vegetarian diet for four months reported some improvement in rheumatoid arthritis, including less pain and better functional capacity, in a Swedish experiment. The diet excluded meat, fish, eggs, and dairy products, strong spices, preservatives, alcohol, tea and coffee. Refined sugar, corn flour and salt were not used or used sparingly.

Source: L. Skoldstam, "Fasting and Vegan Diet in Rheumatoid Arthritis," *Scandinavian Journal of Rheumatology* 15(2):219-21, 1987.

• Fat-free diets have produced complete remissions in six patients with rheumatoid arthritis. Doctors at Wayne State University in Detroit reported that when a low-calorie, low-fat diet in which chicken, cheese, safflower oil, beef, and coconut oil were eliminated, stiffness and swelling of joints disappeared within days. Patients remained symptom free for up to fourteen months, only to experience short-term recurrences within usually 24 to 48 hours of eating foods which were high in fat. "We conclude that dietary fats in amounts normally eaten in the American diet cause the inflammatory joint changes seen in rheumatoid arthritis."

Source: Charles P. Lucas and Lawrence Power, "Dietary Fat Aggravates Active Rheumatoid Arthritis," Department of Medicine, Wayne State University, Detroit, Michigan, 1989.

85. Asthma

Twenty-five patients with bronchial asthma who were put on a strict vegetarian diet showed 71 percent improvement within four months and 92 percent improvement after one year. The experimental diet avoided meat, dairy food, eggs, and fish, as well as sugar, chocolate, salt, and other foods.

Source: O. Lindahl et al., "Vegan Diet Regimen with Reduced Medication in the Treatment of Bronchial Asthma," *Journal of Asthma* 22:45-55, 1985.

86. Bacterial Infection

• An American marine biologist noticed the lack of bacteria in penguin intestines and held the antibiotic qualities of seaweed responsible.

Source: J. M. N. Sieburth, *Sciences* 132:676, 1960.

• Test-tube studies have found that seaweed extract is as effective as antibiotic drugs against common food-poisoning bacteria such as *Staphylococcus aureus* and *Streptococcus pyogenes* and *E. coli*; the fungus *Candida albicans*; and a bacterium associated with causing pneumonia.

Source: O. H. McConnell in H. A. Hoppe et al., *Marine Algae in Pharmaceutical Science* (New York: DeGruyter, 1979).

87. Burn Injuries

Sesame oil is the key ingredient in a new Chinese ointment that aids in the healing of burn injuries. Chinese doctors reported that the herbal compound MEBO ("moist, exposed burn ointment") resulted in dramatic improvement in severely burned patients after treatment. Altogether some 50,000 patients have healed unusually quickly when tested with the substance.

Source: Judy Foreman, "New Chinese Ointment May Aid in the Healing of Burn Injuries," *Boston Globe*, November 23, 1990.

88. Cataracts

Blindness due to cataracts afflicts 50 million persons worldwide. In the U.S. over 541,000 cataract operations are performed annually at a cost of almost $4 billion. Older people who eat a lot of vegetables, fruits, and other nutritious foods have a lower risk of developing cataracts, the leading cause of blindness, according to doctors at Brigham and Women's Hospital in Boston. Studies of 1380 people forty to seventy-nine years old showed that those who received nutritional supplements of vitamins A, B, C, and E found in garden vegetables were 37 percent less likely to have cataracts.

Source: M. Christina Leske and Leo T. Chylack, *Archives of Opthalmology*, February, 1991.

89. Cirrhosis of the Liver

Cirrhosis is the fourth leading cause of death among urban Americans aged 25 to 65. Lecithin, a soybean extract, can delay and possibly prevent cirrhosis of the liver caused by alcohol consumption, according to researchers. In ten-year studies with baboons, scientists in New York found that diets supplemented with about three tablespoons of soy lecithin daily protected the monkeys from scarring and development of cirrhosis. The scientists concluded that this nutritional factor might also be of benefit in humans suffering from alcohol-related liver diseases. Lecithin is found in whole form in miso, tempeh, and other soyfoods.

Source: Charles S. Lieber et al., "Attentuation of Alcohol-Induced Hepatic Fibrosis by Polyunsaturated Lecithin," *Heptology* 12:1390-98, 1990.

90. Colds and Flu

In the Far East, medicinal foods have traditionally been used to help relieve coughs, colds, flu, fatigue, headache, and other symptoms. These include umeboshi plum, kuzu root, and ginger root. Scientists have found that the citric acid in umeboshi serves to neutralize and eliminate lactic acid in the body and that picric acid stimulates the liver and kidneys to cleanse the blood. Powdered kuzu, or kudzu root, also effectively offsets an acidic condition. It is customarily taken in hot bancha tea or water with a little bit of umeboshi and natural soy sauce. Ginger, grated and dissolved in tea, shows an intense anti-cough effect, lowers fever, and reduces pain.

Sources: Moriyasu Ushio, M.D., *The Secrets of the Ume* (Magalia, Ca.: Happiness Press, 1988); William Shurtleff and Akiko Aoyagi, *The Book of Kudzu* (Garden City Park, N.Y.: Avery Publishing Group, 1985); *American Health*, May, 1988.

91. Colitis

A diet high in refined carbohydrates has been associated with ulcerative colitis, non-occlusive ischemic colitis, diverticular disease, and irritable bowel syndrome. A British researcher suggested that eating sugar, white flour, and other simple sugars reduces fecal bulk, allowing intense muscle spasms to occur.

Source: D. S. Grimes, "Refined Carbohydrate, Smooth-Muscle Spasm and Disease of the Colon," *Lancet* 1:395-97, 1976.

92. Diabetes

Each year about a half million new cases of diabetes are diagnosed in the U.S. There are two types: Type 1 or insulin-dependent diabetes mellitus (IDDM) and Type II or noninsulin dependent diabetes mellitus (NIDDM). Formerly these were known as juvenile-onset and adult-onset diabetes respectively. IDDM affects .3 percent of the American population and NIDDM 2.4 percent. Among those 65 and over, about 9 percent have diabetes. Diabetes is particularly associated with the consumption of sugar, white flour, and other refined carbohydrates.

• In 1979 the American Diabetes Association revised its dietary recommendations, recommending that "carbohydrate intake should usually account for 50-60 percent of total energy intake," with "glucose and glucose containing disaccharides (sucrose, lactose) . . . restricted." In addition, the guidelines recommended that "whenever acceptable to the patient, natural foods containing unrefined carbohydrate with fiber should be substituted for highly refined carbohydrates, which are low in fiber" and "dietary sources of fat that are high in saturated fatty acids and foods containing cholesterol should be restricted."

Source: "Principles of Nutrition and Dietary Recommendations for Individuals with Diabetes Mellitus: 1979," *Journal of the American Dietetic Association* 75:527-30.

• Desert plants appear to have protected Native Americans from diabetes before their exposure to modern foods. A study of ancestral diets among the Pima Indians of Arizona shows that a return to mesquite pods, acorns, white and yellow tepary beans, lima beans, and a traditional strain of corn long cultivated by the tribe significantly lowered insulin production and blood sugar levels after meals compared with diets high in potatoes and white bread.

About half of all present-day Pimas over age thirty-five have diabetes. This is the highest incidence of the disease in the world and has been associated with their shift to a modern diet of sugary and fatty foods. The researchers concluded that the benefits of the Pimas' traditional grains, beans, and other foods extended beyond tribal boundaries and would be beneficial for the health of modern people as a whole.

Sources: R. Cowen, "Seeds of Protection," *Science News* 137:350-51, 1990 and Jane Brody, "Arizona Indians Reclaim Ancient Foods," *New York Times*, May 21, 1991.

Nutrients Lost in Refining Whole Wheat			
Nutrient	**Loss (%)**	**Nutrient**	**Loss (%)**
Thiamine (B1)	77.1	Sodium	78.3
Riboflavin (B2)	80.0	Chromium	40.0
Niacin	80.8	Manganese	85.8
Vitamin B6	71.8	Iron	75.6
Panthothenic acid	50.0	Cobalt	88.5
Vitamin E	86.3	Copper	67.9
Calcium	60.0	Zinc	77.7
Phosphorous	70.9	Selenium	15.9
Magnesium	84.7	Molybdenum	48.0
Potassium	77.0		
Source: American Journal of Clinical Nutrition, 1971			

• In Yemen, diabetes was virtually unknown among the Jewish minority. However, when they moved to Israel and adopted the modern diet and lifestyle, incidence of the disease rose to that prevailing in Israel. Kurdish immigrants also experienced the same pattern.

"The change which both communities underwent, as a result of their immigration to Israel," the researcher concluded, "is the transition from an 'oriental' to a 'Western' environment" in which diet may play a central role.

Source: A. M. Cohen, "Effect of Change in Environment on the Prevalence of Diabetes among Yemenite and Kurdish Communities," *Israel Medical Journal* 19:137-42, 1960.

• In tests of a high-fiber complex carbohydrates diet on thirteen diabetic men, aged thirty to thirty-five, five of the men taking oral hypoglycemics were able to discontinue them, four more were able to stop their insulin therapies, and all the others showed some reduction in blood glucose and cholesterol levels. "Every patient that we have treated with the HCF diet has gained some improvement in his or her diabetes. . . we have been able to discontinue insulin therapy in eighteen out of twenty patients taking less than 25 units per day . . . [the HCF diets] lower insulin needs by an average of 25 percent," according to James Anderson, a professor of medicine and clinical nutrition who directs a diabetes program at the Veterans Administration Hospital in Lexington, Kentucky.

Source: James Anderson, M.D., *Diabetes: A Practical New Guide to Healthy Living* (New York: Arco, 1981), pp. 97-98.

• In an Oregon study, six borderline diabetics were put on a macrobiotic diet for thirty days. Excluding the one obese subject, the researchers reported a significant drop in cholesterol levels from a mean of 140 to 110. The subjects were primarily lacto-ovo-vegetarians, accounting for their low cholesterol levels to begin with. A control group of ten macrobiotic subjects showed average cholesterol levels consistent with the Harvard Medical School findings in the mid-1970s.

Source: Mark Mead, "In Search of the Sweet Life: A Dietary Approach to Diabetes Mellitus," Reed College Biology Thesis, in cooperation with the Oregon Health Sciences University, 1984.

93. Diverticulosis

Diverticulosis can be prevented and relieved with a high fiber diet. In a study of sixty-two diverticulosis patients put on a high-fiber diet, 85 percent experienced complete disappearance of their symptoms.

Source: P. Berman and J. B. Kirsner, "Current Knowledge of Diverticular Diseases of the Colon," *American Journal of Digestive Diseases* 17:741-59, 1972.

94. Gallbladder Disease

Vegetarian women had half as many gall stones as women eating the standard modern diet in a study of over 700 women, aged forty to sixty-nine, over several years. Researchers at Oxford University in England concluded that nonvegetarians had nearly twice the risk of developing gall stones and suggested that this was probably the result of the vegetarian women eating more fiber and less fat. "[T]hese data suggest that some dietary factor associated with vegetarianism affords a strong, independent protective effect against this common condition and results in appreciable morbidity in middle aged and elderly women."

Source: F. Pixley et al., "Effect of Vegetarianism on Development of Gall Stones in Women," *British Medical Journal* 291:11-12, 1985.

95. Hearing Loss

A study of over 1400 persons with inner ear symptoms found that when they were given nutritional counseling and put on diets low in saturated fat and high in whole grain cereals and breads, hearing improved. The diets also encouraged vegetable consumption and fruit in place of sugar-sweetened desserts and pastries. Salty foods were avoided as was adding salt to food at the table.

"The response to dietary management is dramatic in most patients," researchers at the West Virginia University School of Medicine reported. "With the otologic patient, dizziness clears promptly and the sensation of pressure in the ears and head is quickly relieved, along with associated headache. Hearing improves or stabilizes, evident in the pure tone audiogram and in the speech discrimination scores. Tinnitus often lessens in severity and sometimes even disappears . . . General health also greatly improves, and elevated blood pressure often returns to normal. The patients have more energy and are free from headaches, their arthritic symptoms improve, and they often sleep better."

Source: J. T. Spencer, "Hyperlipoproteinemia, Hyperinsulinism, and Meniere's Disease," *Southern Medical Journal* 74:1194-97, 1981.

96. Hemorrhoids

In South Africa, whites have high hemorrhoid rates, while blacks rarely experience the condition at all. Researchers have associated hemorrhoids with the whites' diet high in fat and low in fiber and protection from hemorrhoids with the blacks' diet high in fiber and low in fat.

Source: D. Burkitt, "Varicose Veins, Deep Vein Thrombosis and Hemorrhoids: Epidemiology and Suggested Aetiology," *British Medical Journal* 2:556, 1972.

97. Hepatitis

A low-sugar diet may be beneficial to persons suffering from hepatitis. In clinical studies, twenty-one normal men ate the standard American diet with about 25 to 30 percent sucrose for eighteen days and an experimental diet containing less than 10 percent sucrose for twelve days. Levels of transaminase and triglycerides in the blood rose while on the high-sugar diet and returned to normal on the low-sugar diet, suggesting that sugar be reduced or avoided to help protect against hepatitis.

Source: K. P. Porikos and T. B. van Itallie, "Diet-Induced Changes in Serum Transaminase and Triglyceride Levels in Healthy Adult Men," *American Journal of Medicine* 75:624, 1983.

98. Hiatus Hernia

Hiatus hernia in a "characteristically 'Western' disease" caused by a refined diet. "Hiatus hernia seems to be rare in developing countries and almost unknown in communities who have departed little from their traditional way of life," noted two British researchers. "One of us (P.A.J.) did not see a single case of hiatus hernia or esophageal stricture due to reflux esophagitis in an African during seven years as the sole thoracic surgeon in Uganda."

The scientists suggested that the main cause is increased intra-abdominal pressures as a result of eliminating hardened stools from eating meat and other animal food. In Western countries, the average transit time of bowel movements is nearly twice that of people living in native societies. The stools are also harder, more compacted, and weigh about half as much as normal.

Source: D. P. Burkitt and P. A. James, "Low-Residue Diets and Hiatus Hernia," *Lancet* 2:128-30, 1973.

99. Intestinal Disorders

Fermented foods, especially miso, shoyu, tempeh, natto, and other soy products, but also traditionally made pickles and sauerkraut, offer many health benefits such as better food assimilation and the establishment of a beneficial intestinal microflora. A medical researcher at East Carolina University reports that the *Lactobacillus* in these foods can inhibit the action of pathogenic bacteria in the intestines. For example, during World War II, prisoners of war in the Pacific who ate tempeh were observed to be less affected by dysentery, a tropical disease. By reducing harmful bacteria in the digestive tract, fermented foods can reduce the risk to colon cancer and a variety of intestinal disorders. "The inclusion of these fermented foods into one's diet adds a variety of delicious tastes and flavors that complement a vegetable based diet and are excellent sources of many nutrients," the investigator concluded.

Iron Content in Various Foods			
Whole Grains	**mg***	**Sea Vegetables**	**mg***
Buckwheat	3.1	Arame	1.5
Millet	6.8	Dulse	1.6
Oats	4.6	Hijiki	3.2
Soba	5.0	Kombu	1.9
Whole Wheat	3.1	Nori	5.6
Beans		Wakame	1.3
Azuki Beans	4.8	**Seeds**	
Chickpeas	6.9	Pumpkin Seeds	3.2
Lentils	6.8	Sesame Seeds	3.0
Soybeans	7.0	Sunflower Seeds	2.4
Tempeh	5.0	**Animal Food**	
Leafy Vegetables		Milk	0.1
Beet Greens	3.3	Beef	3.6
Dandelion Greens	3.1	Chicken	1.6
Mustard Greens	3.0	Egg Yolk	6.3
Parsley	6.2	Beef Liver	6.5
Spinach	3.1	Oyster	5.5

*Figures are per 100 grams (3.5 oz) except seeds (1 tablespoon) and sea vegetables (1/4 cup, cooked). US RDA varies from 10-18 mg/daily.

Source: U.S.D.A. and Japan Nutritionist Association

Source: W. W. Truslow, "Lactobacillus and Fermented Foods," *Journal of Holistic Medicine* 8:36-46, 1986.

100. Infectious Diseases

In a study of plague and other human diseases, a historian concluded that nearly all of the distinctive infectious diseases of civilization have been transferred to human populations from animal herds used primarily for food. "Measles, for example, is probably related to rinderpest and/or canine distemper; smallpox is certainly connected closely with cowpox and with a cluster of other animal infections; influenza is shared by humans and hogs." The researcher noted that today humans share twenty-six diseases with poultry, forty-two with pigs, forty-six with sheep and goats, and fifty with cattle.

Source: William H. McNeill, *Plagues and Peoples* (Garden City, N.Y.: Anchor Press/Doubleday, 1976), p. 51.

101. Iron Deficiency

Traditional naturally processed soy products produce more iron than soyfoods that are processed in modern ways. South African researchers report that the bio-availability of unprocessed soy flour that is commonly used in modern foods was poor and could inhibit iron absorption from other foods in the diet. In comparison, miso, tempeh, natto, and other traditionally processed soy products were found to have greater bioavailability.

Source: Bruce J. Macfarlane et al., "Effect of Traditonal Oriental Soy Products on Iron Absorption," *American Journal of Clinical Nutrition* 51:873-80, 1990.

102. Kidney Disease

• In a study designed to measure the effect of a low animal protein diet on the risk of urinary stone disease, researchers in Britain reported that a nation-wide survey of vegetarians in the U.K. showed that the prevalence of kidney stone formation was 40 to 60 percent of the general population. "The findings support the hypothesis that a diet low in animal protein reduces the risk of urinary stone formation," the scientists concluded.

Source: W. G. Robertson et al., "The Prevalence of Urinary Stone Disease in Vegetarians," *European Urology* 8:334-39, 1982.

• Increase of fiber and reduction of sugar, refined carbohydrates, and animal protein significantly reduced the excretion of calcium, oxalate, and uric acid in the urine. Researchers recommended this dietary approach as a way of treating and managing kidney stones.

Source: P. N. Rao et al., "Dietary Management of Urinary Risk Factors in Renal Stone Formers," *British Journal of Urology* 54:578-83, 1982.

• In 1981, Guillermo Asis, M.D., a young medical doctor in Boston, developed a kidney-stone attack. Asis attributed the cause to a diet high in beef and sugar and low in grains and vegetables in his native Argentina. At the time, he had been studying at the Kushi Institute in Brookline and decided to try a traditional Far Eastern home remedy. "The pain was unbearable," he reported. "While colleagues were ready to administer heavy pain medications and admit me to the hospital for x-rays, I insisted upon only having applications of hot-compress preparations made from the juice of ginger root. I strongly suspect that some doctors thought I was crazy. As it turned out, I felt better than before the attack, with only three applications of the ginger compress during a 48-hour period. And I never had the problem again. I felt truly proud of not having taken even an aspirin or Tylenol during that episode."

Source: Guillermo Asis, M.D., "Awakening to Common Sense," in *Doctors Look at Macrobiotics* (Tokyo & New York: Japan Publications, 1988), pp. 169-76.

103. Migraine Headache

• Five women with chronic migraines were put on an experimental diet which resulted in complete elimination of headache pain in four of the women.

Source: D. R. O'Banion, "Dietary Control of Headache Pain: Five Case Studies," *Journal of Holistic Medicine* 3:140-51, 1981.

• A former medical consultant for the Department of National Health and Welfare in Canada successfully treated her own migraine headache with diet. Dr. Helen V. Farrell reported that she suffered from classical migraines since she was eleven, experiencing scintillating scotomas, dysplasia, transient parasthesias, and vomiting. As she grew older, the headaches were less frequent, and when she discontinued dairy food and exercised regularly they began to disappear altogether. However, in July, 1987, she began to experience a recurrence and decided to treat it with a macrobiotic home remedy.

"By the time I got home twenty minutes later," she reported, "I could barely see, and the pounding migraine pain was just starting. I headed straight for the pantry and the umeboshi plum paste. I had been reading about this condiment and its 'contractiveness,' so I thought I would experiment and see if it worked or not. After about two teaspoons and within two minutes, the visual symptoms disappeared dramatically. I couldn't believe it!" Every twenty minutes, she continued eating a little more umeboshi and within two hours

"I got up, feeling completely normal with no headache, nausea, or tingling."

Dr. Farrell, who specializes in treating female complaints, has successfully introduced many of her patients to a macrobiotic diet. She reports that it is particularly effective in treating premenstrual syndrome.

Source: Helen V. Farrell, M.D., "PMS Is Not PMS," in *Doctors Look at Macrobiotics* (Tokyo & New York: Japan Publications, 1988), pp. 177-91.

104. Motion Sickness

Medical researchers report that ginger root, especially in powdered form, is beneficial for treating motion sickness. In the Far East, umeboshi plums also have traditionally been used for motion sickness, as well as nausea, stomach upset, and digestive problems.

Sources: J. Backon, "Ginger: Inhibition of Thromboxane Synthetase and Stimulaton of Prostacyclin: Relevance for Medicine and Psychiatry," *Medical Hypotheses* 20:271-78, 1986 and Michio Kushi and Marc Van Cauwenberghe, M.D., *Macrobiotic Home Remedies* (Tokyo and New York: Japan Publications, 1987).

105. Multiple Sclerosis

In a review of treating cases of multiple sclerosis with a low-fat diet for more than twenty years, Roy L. Swank, M.D., of the Divison of Neurology, University of Oregon Medical School, reported that in 146 patients monitored, there was a 70 percent decrease in the relapse rate of MS the first year and a subsequent additional decrease of 25 percent in the succeeding five years. The death rate in MS patients on the usual high-fat diet was three to four times higher than in patients in this study. The therapeutic diet consisted of 25 to 29 percent fats and oils and calories averaged 1788 for women and 2164 for men — both well below the national average. Fish was recommended instead of meat, and most patients increased their intake of vegetables, fruits, and other plant-quality foods. "The course of disease in these patients was less rapidly progressive than in untreated cases available in the literature for comparison," Dr. Swank concluded. "There was a significant reduction in the death rate, in the frequency and severity of exacerbations, and in the rate at which patients became unable to walk and work. If treated early in the disease, before significant disability had developed, a high percentage of cases remained unchanged for up to twenty years. When treated later in disease, the disease usually continued to be slowly progressive. Patients who consumed the least amount of fat and the largest amounts of fluid oils deteriorated less than those who consumed more fat and less oil."

Source: R. L. Swank, "Multiple Sclerosis: Twenty Years on Low Fat Diet," *Archives of Neurology* 23:460-74, 1970.

106. Obesity

"Obesity and diabetes mellitus . . . usually emerge together about the same time in any community that is becoming affluent, wherein the wealthy are able to consume more fat, oil, sugar, meat, wine and beer, also refined cereals, such as white bread and white rice. Little is known concerning the ancient date when, in India and China, rice began to be [processed] to produce low fiber white rice . . . . Perhaps this explains why diabetes mellitus emerges as a common disease at an early date in India and China."

Source: H. Trowell and D. Burkitt, editors, *Western Diseases: Their Emergence and Prevention*, (Cambridge, Mass: Harvard University Press, 1981), p. 24.

107. Osteoporosis

Osteoporosis, characterized by thinning of the bones and susceptibility to fracture, commonly affects elderly people in modern society and gets progressively worse with age. Conventional medicine has treated this disease with increased consumption of dairy food and other foods high in calcium and calcium supplements. Current research suggests that excessive animal protein, not lack of dietary calcium, is the primary cause of this degenerative ill.

• The Inuit (Eskimo) have the highest osteoporosis rates in the world. In a study of 217 children, 89 adults, and 107 elderly Inuit in Alaska, researchers found that they had lower bone mineral content, onset of bone loss at an earlier age, and development of bone thinning with a greater intensity than white Americans. The scientists attributed the greater degeneration to the acidic effects of the Inuits' high meat diet.

Sources: R. Mazess and W. Mather, "Bone Mineral Content of North Alaskan Eskimos," *American Journal of Clinical Nutrition* 27:916-25, 1974.

Calcium Content in Various Foods			
Leafy Green Vegetables	**mg***	**Sea Vegetables**	**mg***
Broccoli	246	Agar-Agar	100
Collard Greens	177	Arame	146
Daikon Greens	80	Dulse	137
Dandelion Greens	74	Hijiki	152
Kale	103	Kombu	76
Mustard Greens	97	Nori	100
Parsley	61	Wakame	130
Spinach	83	**Grains & Seeds**	
Turnip Greens	126	Buckwheat	57
Watercress	90	Sesame Seeds	331
Beans and Products		Sweet Almonds	81
Azuki Beans	37	Sunflower Seeds	40
Chickpeas	75	Brazil Nuts	53
Kidney Beans	70	Hazel Nuts	60
Navy Beans	95	**Dairy Food**	
Soybeans	131	Milk	288
Miso	40	Eggs	27
Natto	103	Goat's Milk	315
Tempeh	142	Cheese, various	100-350
Tofu	128	Yogurt	272

*Figures are for average servings: greens (1/2 cup cooked); beans (1 cup, cooked), sea vegetables (1/4 cup, cooked); grain (1 cup, cooked), seeds and nuts (1 tablespoon); dairy (1 cup, 1 large egg, or 1 slice cheece). US RDA varies from 800 - 1200 mg/daily.

Source: U.S.D.A. and Japan Nutritionist Association

• A Michigan State study found that by age 65, the average woman who ate meat had lost one-third of her skeletal structure. Meanwhile, vegetarian woman of comparable age had less than half the bone loss and were more active, less likely to break bones, maintained erect postures, and healed bones more quickly.

Source: F. Ellis et al., "Incidence of Osteoporosis in Vegetarians and Omnivores," *American Journal of Clinical Nutrition* 27:916, 1974.

• Researchers from Creighton University in Omaha, Nebraska, and Purdue University in West Lafayette, Indiana, reported that the calcium in kale is readily absorbed by the body and more efficiently than the calcium contained in milk. In studies of eleven women, the absorption of calcium from 300 mg. of kale averaged .409, while from a similar amount of milk calcium absorption averaged .321.

"We interpret our findings as evidence of good bioavailability for kale calcium and probably for the loss of low-oxalate vegetable greens as well," the researchers concluded. Other greens they listed included broccoli, turnip, mustard, and collard greens.

Source: Robert P. Heaney and Connie M. Weaver, "Calcium Absorption from Kale," *American Journal of Clinical Nutrition* 51: 656-57,1990.

108. Parkinson's Disease

A low protein diet may help persons with Parkinson's disease. Experimental studies of eleven patients who had Parkinson's disease for six to twenty years and who were put on a low protein diet resulted in reduced movement fluctuations and the less need for drugs. Foods high in protein that were avoided included all meats, egg white, gelatin, dairy food, beans and nuts, and chocolate and pastries. Recommended foods included cereals, toast, all green and yellow vegetables, fresh and dried fruit, sherbert, condiments, and fluids. Researchers at Yale University reported that all adjuvant therapy could be discontinued as the subjects experienced improvement. "On this diet, patients can predictably expect daytime mobility, thus permitting near-normal function and independence at home or on the job."

Source: J. H. Pincus and K. Barry, "Influence of Dietary Protein on Motor Flucuations in Parkinson's Disease," *Archives of Neurology* 44:270-72, 1987.

109. Premenstrual Syndrome (PMS)

• A survey found that women with anxiety symptoms associated with PMS, including nervous tension, mood swings, irritability, anxiety, and insomnia, ate two and a half times as much sugar as women without PMS or with mild cases. Dairy and caffeine intake have also been associated with PMS in other studies.

Sources: G.E. Abraham, "Magnesium Deficiency in Premenstrual Tension," *Magnesium Bulletin* 1:68-73, 1982.

• MIT researchers reported that women consuming a diet high in complex carbohydrates and low in protein showed "improved depression, tension, anger, confusion, sadness, fatigue, alertness, and calmness" before the onset of menstruation in comparison to women with severe PMS eating the usual diet high in refined carbohydrates and fat. Besides sweets, the women suffering from PMS consumed more calories and more snack foods. Evidence was found that they intuitively tried to generate positive moods by ingesting more carbohydrates such as bread, rolls, and pasta and avoiding foods rich in protein.

Source: Judith J. Wurtman et al., "Effect of Nutrient Intake on Premenstrual Depression," *American Journal of Obstetrics and Gynecology* 161:1228-34, 1989.

• A new medical textbook on reproductive health and disorders recommends a high-fiber, low-fat diet to help prevent or reduce PMS. "Diet throughout the month, and especially during the premenstrual interval, should be high in complex carbohydrates and moderate in protein (emphasizing alternatives to red meat), but low in refined sugar and salt (sodium), with regular, small meals throughout the day." The authors further recommended that "women should reduce or eliminate their consumption of tea, coffee, caffeine-containing beverages, chocolate, and alcohol, and stop smoking."

Source: Robert A. Hatcher et al., "Menstrual Problems," *Contraceptive Technology 1990-1992* (New York: Irvington, 1990).

110. Rheumatism

Common nightshade vegetables may be associated with rheumatism and arthritis. In an experiment in which 5000 arthritis patients avoided white potatoes, peppers, tomato, eggplant, and tobacco, 70 percent reported progressive relief from aches and pains and from some disfigurement over seven years.

Source: N. F. Childers, "A Relationship of Arthritis to the *Solanaceae* (Nightshades)," *Journal of the International Academy of Preventive Medicine*, November, 1982, pp. 31-37.

111. Tooth Decay

In a National Health Survey for 1971-73, Americans of both sexes and all ages from one to seventy-four had an average of thirteen decayed, missing, and filled permanent teeth. An estimated 15 percent of adults had lost all their permanent teeth. "Until the 1970s, caries was most prevalent (affecting 95 percent of the population) in developed countries," researchers noted, "especially in those with diets high in refined carbohydrates. The only exception occurred during and just after World War II, when the prevalence rates of caries dropped precipitously, although temporarily, in children living in Europe."

Source: National Academy of Sciences, *Diet and Health* (Washington, D.C.: National Academy Press), 1989, p. 127.

112. Ulcers

In a random case-control study of seventy-three persons with recently healed duodenal ulcers, the group put on high-fiber diet consisting of whole grain bread, soft oats, barley, or wheat, and plenty of vegetables experienced about half as much relapse after six months as the group eating the usual diet. Researchers in Oslo, Norway, reported that 80 percent of the persons who ate the least amount of whole grains, cereal products, or vegetables developed new ulcers. "A diet rich in fiber may, therefore, protect against duodenal ulceration," the investigators concluded.

Ulcers have also been associated with frequent milk consumption, hot spicy foods, alcohol, and sugar.

Source: A. Rydning et al., "Prophylactic Effect of Dietary Fiber in Duodenal Ulcer Disease," *Lancet* 2:736-39, 1982.

113. Zinc Deficiency

Zinc deficiencies are increasingly common in pregnant mothers, teenagers, and in the elderly. They have been associated in medical studies with learning disabilities, infertility, immunodepression, sickle-cell anemia, slower healing of wounds, and other disorders.

Whole sources of zinc include brown rice, barley, whole wheat, rye, oats, and other whole cereal grains; nuts; sunflower and pumpkin seeds; sea vegetables; lentils and peas; watercress and parsley.

Sources: National Academy of Sciences, *Diet and Health* (Washington, D.C.: National Academy Press, 1989) and Michio Kushi and Martha Cottrell, *AIDS, Macrobiotics, and Natural Immunity* (Tokyo and New York, Japan Publications, 1990).

Scientific Studies and Medical Reports Associating Diet and Degenerative Disease

	Coronary Heart Disease	High Blood Pressure	Breast Cancer	Colon Cancer	Lung Cancer	Stomach Cancer	Other Cancers	Radiation Sickness	AIDS	Diabetes	Osteo-porosis
Beneficial											
Whole Grains	•	•	•	•	•	•	•	•	•	•	•
Beans	•		•	•			•		•	•	•
Miso	•	•	•			•	•	•	•		•
Tofu	•					•					•
Vegetables	•		•	•	•	•	•		•	•	•
Leafy Green				•	•		•	•			•
Yellow/Orange	•				•		•	•			
Sea Vegetables	•	•	•				•	•	•		•
Fruit	•			•							
Sea Salt		•					•	•	•		
Polyunsat. Fat/Oil	•	•	•	•	•	•	•	•	•	•	•
Harmful											
Meat	•	•	•	•	•	•	•		•	•	•
Poultry	•	•	•	•	•		•		•	•	•
Eggs	•	•	•	•	•		•		•		•
Dairy	•	•	•	•	•		•		•		•
Sugar		•	•				•		•	•	
White Flour/Rice			•	•		•	•	•	•	•	
Refined Salt		•				•		•			
Saturated Fat/Oil	•	•	•	•		•		•	•	•	•

6

Protecting Against Radiation

In August, 1945, following the atomic bombing of Nagasaki, Dr. Aki-zuki saved the lives of all of his patients from radiation sickness by giving them brown rice, miso soup, land and sea vegetables, and other macrobiotic-quality foods. Survivors in Hiroshima also experienced similar benefits. In the 1960s, scientists in Canada started experimenting with some of these foods in the quest for an antidote to fallout from worldwide atomic testing and showed that common seaweeds offered effective protection. In the 1980s, scientists in Hiroshima began a series of experiments with miso soup that have also demonstrated a measure of immunity. Following the nuclear accident at Chernobyl in 1986, thousands of Europeans increased their intake of these foods, and in the early 1990s, Soviet doctors began treating children and adults exposed to radioactivity with miso, sea vegetables, and other beneficial foods.

114. Diet and the Atomic Bombing of Nagasaki

In August, 1945, at the time of the atomic bombing of Japan, Tatsuichiro Akizuki, M.D., was director of the Department of Internal Medicine at St. Francis's Hospital in Nagasaki. Most patients in the hospital, located one mile from the center of the blast, survived the initial effects of the bomb, but soon after came down with symptoms of radiation sickness from the fallout that had been released. Dr. Akizuki fed his staff and patients a strict macrobiotic diet of brown rice, miso and tamari soy sauce soup, wakame and other sea vegetables, Hokkaido pumpkin, and sea salt and prohibited the consumption of sugar and sweets. As a result, he saved everyone in his hospital, while many other survivors in the city perished from radiation sickness.

"I gave the cooks and staff strict orders that they should make unpolished whole-grain rice balls, adding some salt to them, prepare strong miso soup for each meal, and never use sugar. When they didn't follow my orders, I scolded them without mercy, 'Never take sugar. Sugar will destroy your blood!'. . .

"This dietary method made it possible for me to remain alive and go on working vigorously as a doctor. The radioactivity may not have been a fatal dose, but thanks to this method, Brother Iwanaga, Reverend Noguchi, Chief Nurse Miss Murai, other staff members and in-patients, as well as myself, all kept on living on the lethal ashes of the bombed ruins. It was thanks to this food that all of us could work for people day after day, overcoming fatigue or symptoms of atomic disease and survive the disaster free from severe symptoms of radioactivity."

Sources: Tatsuichiro Akizuki, M.D., *Nagasaki 1945* (London: Quartet Books, 1981); Tatsuichiro Akizuki, "How We Survived Nagasaki," *East West Journal*, December 1980.

115. Diet and Radiation Sickness in Hiroshima

In 1945, Sawako Hirago was a ten-year-old school girl in Hiroshima. In the atomic bombing on August 6, she was exposed to severe radiation that burned her face, head, and legs. The burned parts swelled up nearly three times normal. In the hospital, doctors feared for her recovery because one-third of her body was burned. Her mother gave her palm healing therapy over the abdomen every night, and she ate the only food available, two rice balls and two daikon radish pickles each day. Inside the rice balls was umeboshi (pickled salted plums).

Although the medical doctors gave up on her, Sawako survived, "My mother didn't show me a mirror until I was cured. However, I was able to see my hands and leg which were very dirty and had a bad, rotten smell. On the rotten spots there were always flies. When the skin healed, I broke it because it was itchy; finally it became a keloidal condition. I didn't see my face until it was finally cured. However, sores remained on my nose and pus remained on my chest. My hands and chest had masses of skin which remained until I was twenty."

Because of her disfiguration, she was ridiculed, nicknamed "Hormone Short," and told she could never marry or have children. After completing school, she became a high school physics teacher and met a young chemistry teacher who ate very simply. The couple married and attended lectures by George Ohsawa, the founder of modern macrobiotics in Japan, and he said that only people practicing macrobiotics would survive a future nuclear war.

After talking with Mr. Ohsawa, Sawako gave up the modern, refined food which she had been eating since her survival and started eating brown rice and other foods. To her surprise, her problems started to clear up, including anemia, leukemia, low blood pressure, falling hair, and bleeding from the nose. Within two months, she was elated, "My face became beautiful."

Sawako went on to have seven healthy children and raised all of them on brown rice, miso soup, vegetables, seaweed, and other healthy food.

Source: Sawako Hiraga, "How I Survived the Atomic Bomb," *The Macrobiotic,* November/December 1979.

116. Sea Vegetables and Strontium-90

• Scientists at the Gastro-Intestinal Research Laboratory at McGill University in Montreal, Canada, reported that a substance derived from the sea vegetable kelp could reduce by 50 to 80 percent the amount of radioactive strontium absorbed through the intestine. Stanley Skoryna, M.D., said that in animal experiments sodium alginate obtained from brown algae permitted calcium to be normally absorbed through the intestinal wall while binding most of the strontium. The sodium alginate and strontium were subsequently excreted from the body. The experiments were designed to devise a method to counteract the effects of nuclear fallout and radiation.

Source: S. C. Skoryna et al., "Studies on Inhibition of Intestinal Absorption of Radioactive Strontium," *Canadian Medical Association Journal* 91:285-88, 1964.

• Canadian researchers reported that sea vegetables contained a polysaccharide substance that selectively bound radioactive strontium and helped eliminate it from the body. In laboratory experi-

Inhibitory Effects of Seaweed Alginates on the Intestinal Absorption of Radioactive Strontium	
	Reduction of Bone Uptake (%)
Species of Seaweed	Strontium
A. Extracted from dry seaweeds	
Ascophyllum nodosum	58
Fucus endentatus	51
Fucus vesiculosus (Bladderwrack)	70
Laminaria digitata, blades (Kombu)	44
Laminaria spp., unidentified small plant (Kombu)	57
Nereocystis leutkeana, blades	44
B. Extracted from wet seaweeds	
Alaria marginata (a)	3
Egregia menziessi	74
Hedophyllum sessile (a)	35
Hedophyllum sessile (b)	26
Laminaria spp., unidentified narrow blades (Kombu)	34
Macrocystis pyrifera (Giant Kelp)	80
Nereocystis leutkeana (a)	69
Pelvetia spp.	50
Postelsia palmaeformis, stipes	26
C. Extracted from acid-treated dry seaweed	
Alaria marginata (b)	60
Costaria costata	63
Laminaria digitata	60
Nereocystis leutkeana (b) (Bull Whip Kelp)	54
Source: Canadian Medical Association Journal, 1968	

ments, sodium alginate prepared from kelp, kombu, and other brown seaweeds off the Atlantic and Pacific coasts was introduced along with strontium and calcium into rats. The reduction of radioactive particles in bone uptake, measured in the femur, reached as high as 80 percent, with little interference with calcium absorption. "The evaluation of biological activity of different marine algae is important because of their practical significance in preventing absorption of radioactive products of atomic fission as well as in their use as possible natural decontaminators."

Source: Y. Tanaka et al., "Studies on Inhibition of Intestinal Absorption of Radio-Active Strontium," *Canadian Medical Association Journal* 99:169-75, 1968.

117. Miso and Radiation

• A team studying atomic bomb radioactivity has found miso is effective in helping to remove radioactive elements from the body and controlling inflammation of organs caused by radioactivity.

In experiments conducted on male and female rats four weeks after birth, radioisotopes of iodine-131 and cesium-134 were injected into the animals' stomachs. Both isotopes are secondary elements produced in nuclear reactor accidents. The iodine-131 isotope is absorbed in the thyroid gland, while the cesium-134 accumulates in muscles and in the intestines.

Researchers at Hiroshima University Medical Center found that there was only half the amount of iodine-131 in the blood of the group fed with miso in contrast to the control group three and six hours after the injections. Lower amounts of radioactive particles were also measured in the kidneys, liver, and spleen.

Although there was no difference in the amount of radioactive cesium in the blood, a high amount of cesium was eliminated from the muscles of the group eating miso.

In other tests of exposure to a half lethal dose of radiation to test the effect of miso on victims of a nuclear explosion, more than 80 percent of the rats from each group died within one week. However, the inflammation of organs commonly seen after exposure to radiation was less for the rats eating miso. Akihiro Ito, head of the Hiroshima University medical team, said that this showed that miso stimulated the body's circulatory and metabolic system.

Source: "Miso Show Promise as Treatment for Radiation," *The Japan Times,* September 27, 1988.

• People who eat miso regularly may be up to five times more resistant to radiation than people not eating miso. This is the conclusion of scientific studies conducted by Kazumitsu Watanabe, professor of cancer and radiation at Hiroshima University's atomic bomb radiation research center.

In laboratory experiments, he tested the cells in the small intestine of mice. These cells absorb nutrients and are particularly sensitive to radiation. They are easily destroyed by radiation. The victims of Hiroshima and Nagasaki suffered from severe cases of diarrhea after the atomic bomb because of massive destruction of these cells.

Forty-nine-week-old mice were given miso as 10 percent of their food for seven days prior to exposure to radiation. Mice were exposed to full body X-rays 1400 to 2400 times stronger than a regular medical X-ray (7-10 curies). Three days later their cells were examined. The loss of cells was less severe in the miso-eating mice than in regular mice. When 9 curies were administered, the gap between miso-eating and regular mice's loss of cells became greater. Ten curies is a lethal dose for humans. When 10 curies were given to miso-eating mice, 60 percent survived, compared to only 9 percent of the mice which did not eat miso.

"I don't know specifically what element in miso is effective," Professor Watanabe told the South Western Japan Conference on the Effects of Radiation. "The small intestines of mice and humans are quite similar. Therefore this study indicates that miso is a preventive measure against radiation."

In other tests at Hiroshima University, it has already been shown that miso has the property of eliminating radiation from the body and can help relieve liver cancer. Plans for further studies include how miso affects cancer of the large intestine and stomach as well as the effect of radiation on blood pressure.

Sources: "Miso Protects Against Radiation," *Yomiuri Shinbun*, July 16, 1990; "People Who Consume Miso Regularly Are More Resistant to Radiation," *Nikan Kogyo Shinbun* (*Daily Business and Technology Newspaper*), July 25, 1990.

• Soviet physicians began incorporating miso soup into the diets of patients suffering from radiation symptoms and cancer. "Miso is helping some of our patients with terminal cancer to survive," reported Lidia Yamchuk, M.D. and Hanif Shaimandarov, M.D., doctors in Cheljabinsk, site of a major nuclear accident. "Their blood (and blood analysis) become better after they began to use miso in their daily food."

Source: Personal communication to Alex Jack, April, 1991.

7

Strengthening Natural Immunity

The spread of AIDS and other immune-deficiency diseases has been increasingly linked with imbalanced diet and lifestyle. In addition to prevention, proper food can help persons recover from serious illness. The pioneer studies — undertaken by medical researchers in Boston and New York — examined a group of young men with AIDS who started a macrobiotic diet. Though some of the men died because their illness was too advanced, others survived, and the group as a whole lived longer than any control group following conventional treatment. Proper food also promises to be beneficial for environmental illness (EI), systemic lupus erythematosus (SLE), Epstein-Barr virus (EBV), cytomegalovirus (CMV), and other sicknesses associated with loss of natural immunity.

118. Macrobiotic AIDS Study

• In 1983 a group of men in New York City with AIDS (Acquired Immuno-deficiency Syndrome) began macrobiotics under the inspiration of Michio Kushi and Lawrence H. Kushi, D.Sc. They hoped to change their blood quality, recover their natural immmunity, and survive this otherwise always fatal illness. In May,1984, a research team led by Elinor N. Levy, Ph.D. and John C. Beldekas, Ph.D. of the Department of Immunology and Microbiology at Boston University's School of Medicine and Martha C. Cottrell, M.D., Director of Student Health at the Fashion Institute of Technology in

New York, began to monitor the blood samples and immune functions of ten men with Kaposi's sarcoma (a usual symptom of AIDS). Preliminary results indicated that most of the men were stabilizing on the diet. "Survival in these men who have received little or no medical treatment appears to compare very favorably with that of KS patients in general. We suggest that physicians and scientists can feel comfortable in allowing patients, particularly those with minimal disease, to go untreated as part of a larger [dietary] study or because non-treatment is the patient's choice."

Source: "Patients with Kaposi Sarcoma Who Opt for No Treatment" [Letter], *Lancet*, July 1985.

• At the International AIDS Conference in Paris in June, 1986, Elinor Levy and associates presented further findings concerning the men with Kaposi's sarcoma who had been practicing macrobiotics. In their conclusions, the researchers noted:

1. Lymphocyte number increases over the first two years from diagnosis with Kaposi's sarcoma in men who are following a macrobiotic diet. A linear regression analysis model predicts that lymphocyte number becomes normal within this two-year period.

2. During this time period the percentage of T4 cells does not change. The percentage of T8 cells possibly decreases.

3. These results compare favorably with those from any of the medical treatments reported.

4. There are several possible explanations for these positive findings including: a) the macrobiotic diet and/or lifestyle is of benefit to men with Kaposi's sarcoma. b) The decision to become and remain macrobiotic selects for men with a better prognosis.

Source: Elinor Levy, J. C. Beldekas, P. H. Black, and L. H. Kushi, "Patients with Kaposi's Sarcoma Who Opt for Alternative Therapy," International AIDS Conference, Paris, France, 1986.

• In further report on the men in the macrobiotic AIDS study, Dr. Levy reported in 1988: "The large majority of subjects reported a decrease in AIDS-related symptoms, particularly fatigue (23/29) and diarrhea (17/19). The lymphocyte number in the subgroup of nineteen subjects with Kaposi's sarcoma alone tended to increase with time after diagnosis. Only two of this group of nineteen lost more than 10 percent of their body weight during their participation in the study which ranged from several months to more than three

LYMPHOCYTE NUMBER Vs. TIME
IN PEOPLE WITH KS [P<.003]

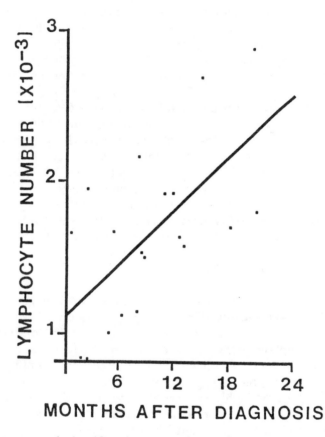

The average calculated lymphocyte number/mm^3 increases from 1122 at diagnosis to 2584 two years later. The calculation is based on all the data points available.

Source: Levy et al., 1986.

years. Nine of the nineteen with KS have died, seven are alive more than three years after diagnosis with KS."
Source: Elinor M. Levy, Letter to the American Cancer Society, March 3, 1988.

• After initial observations, the macrobiotic AIDS test group was expanded to twenty men. "As a group, the men have had significant improvement in their total T-cell numbers, notably in T4 counts, although T4/T8 ratios have not changed significantly," Martha Cottrell reported. "Those with Kaposi's sarcoma have shown the best survival rates, three going five years or longer. The approach has demonstrated effective in managing their condition while minimizing opportunistic infections and use of toxic drugs. They are all working full time and enjoying a quality of life atypical of most AIDS patients. Most of all, they are relatively free of the sense of hopelessness, helplessness, and victimization which tends to take hold of other AIDS patients. Thus the physical benefits — prolonging life and improving the immunocompetence — seems complemented by a range of psychological benefits."
Source: Martha Cottrell, Letter to the American Cancer Society, March 14, 1988. See also Tom Monte, *The Way of Hope* (New York: Warner Books, 1990).

119. AIDS in Africa

One of the most intriguing observations in Africa is the significant correlation beteween AIDS and upper-class status. This strongly suggests a possible association with environmental factors. Urban centers throughout Africa have been increasingly influenced by Western technology, including the typical American diet of refined sugars and flours, meats, eggs, dairy products, food additives, and other foods. In the highly Westernized city of Kinshasa, capital of the Republic of the Congo, this dietary pattern is far more typical of urban people in the upper income bracket.

"It seems plausible that the rapid modernization of Africa's urban population, particularly for the upper class, may have set the stage for compromised immunity and thereby predisposed them to the pathogenic effects of the AIDS virus," concluded Martha Cottrell, M.D. who gave seminars on diet and AIDS in West Africa.

The typical upper-class diet, based on the haute-cuisine of French and Belgian, includes imported red meats, eggs, white sugar, baked white-flour products, dairy, hydrogenated oils, and imported fruits and vegetables. "Heavy reliance on imported products has introduced high levels of artificial preservatives and agricultural chemicals to the urban elite's food supply. Clearly this is not the kind of diet one would expect to support resistance to infectious diseases."

By contrast, the native lower class diet includes locally grown fruit, cassava meal (a starchy root vegetables), avocados, red onions, and small amounts of fish, game, insects. "In sum, the typical diet of low-income Kinshasans is basically low in protein, low in fat, and high in complex carbohydrates and fiber. By nutritional standards, this type of dietary pattern would clearly favor strong immunity."

Source: Michio Kushi and Martha Cottrell, M.D., with Mark Mead, *AIDS, Macrobiotics, and Natural Immunity* (Tokyo & New York: Japan Publications, 1990), pp. 216-17.

120. Saliva and Natural Immunity

When AIDS first appeared in 1981, macrobiotic educator Michio Kushi began recommending thorough chewing as a key dietary measure to help prevent the development of immune deficiency. He noted that the yang, contractive properties of saliva, which is promoted during chewing, could help neutralize the extreme yin, expansive quality of the AIDS virus. Now medical studies for this theory have emerged. Saliva contains substances that prevent the AIDS virus from infecting white-blood cells. In a study, researchers tested saliva from three healthy men, thirty-five, forty, and forty-two years old. Tests indicated the men were not carriers of the AIDS virus and were not known to be at high-risk for infection. In laboratory dishes, the men's saliva prevented the AIDS virus from infecting lymphoctes, a type of white-blood cell that is among the immune system cells attacked by the AIDS virus in the body.

The dental researchers said the finding might help explain why no cases have been documented in which the AIDS virus was transmitted from person to person through saliva such as through kissing or sharing toothbrushes. The scientists concluded that saliva is well known to contain substances that kill bacteria and funguses and so might also be able to block the AIDS virus.

Source: P. C. Fox et al., "Saliva Inhibits HIV-1 Infectivity," *Journal of the American Dental Association* 116:635-37, 1988.

121. Vitamin A, Beta-Carotene, and AIDS

Retinoids (foods and substances high in vitamin A) and carotenoids (foods and substances high in beta-carotene, a precursor to vitamin A) can stimulate some human immune responses, including heightened anti-tumor cell activity, increased natural killer cell response, and activated lymphocytes.

Researchers at the University of Arizona reported that retinoids and carotenoids appear to have different effects on the immune system. Retinoids act on the differentiation processes of immune cells, increasing mitogenesis of lymphocytes and enhancing phagocytosis of monocytes and macrophages as well as acting as anti-oxidants reducing loss of immunological functions due to free radicals. Carotenoids increase T-helper cell numbers and natural killer cells. "Restoring the number of these cells may be useful in acquired immunodeficiency syndromes such as (AIDS) where immune cells are in low numbers and defective in nature," the researchers noted. The scientists recommended that clinical trials begin to study the role of these dietary agents in AIDs patients.

Foods naturally high in these nutrients include orange and yellow vegetables such as carrots, squash, parsnips, and rutabaga.

Source: R. H. Prabhala et al., "Immunomodulation in Humans Caused by Beta-Carotene and Vitamin A," *Nutrition Research* 10:1473-86, 1990.

122. Diet and Natural Immunity

In a review of AIDS research between 1981 and 1990, a senior medical researcher speculated that AIDS may not be caused primarily by a virus but may be the result of immunosuppressive behavior and lifestyle, especially the abuse of drugs and medications and improper diet. Dr. Peter H. Duesberg, professor of molecular and cell biology at the University of California, Berkeley and a pioneer in retrovirus research, concluded that AIDS is not a single infectious disease or syndrome but a set of separate conditions with different risk factors. He cited the use of nitrite inhalants or "poppers" and other aphrodisiac drugs as well as prior use of alcohol, heroin, cocaine, marijuana, valium, and amphetamines as chief causes of loss of natural immunity in the gay community. In Africa, where AIDS is commonly known as "Slim Disease," he noted that it does not appear to be contagious but rather fits the profile of malnutrition, apparently caused in part by modern foods.

The use of AZT, an anti-HIV drug, should be discontinued, he concluded, because it only weakens the immune system. "Doctors should treat each condition separately, and should seek to determine the underlying causes in each individual's case; patients should insist on this approach from their doctors. But perhaps the most useful action for any such patient to take would be the ending of any risk behavior. Unfortunately, no studies have been done, but anecdotal case descriptions exist of AIDS patients who recover after ending drug use, sexual promiscuity, and prophylactic antibiotic use, and who improve their nutritional status." Among the cases cited are thirteen AIDS survivors, including some who practiced macrobiotics, who have lived more than five years since their diagnosis.

Source: Peter H. Duesberg and Bryan J. Ellison, *Policy Review*, Summer, 1990, pp. 40-51.

123. Environmental Illness

In 1974 Sherry A. Rogers, M.D., then a thirty-one-year-old physician, suffered from Environmental Illness. She had ugly red eczema over the lower half of her face, periodic asthma, recurrent sinus problems, wicked migraines, chronic back pain from an old riding injury, and unwarranted exhaustion and depression.

By the early 1980s she was having strong adverse reactions to chemicals such as workmen glueing down a new Formica countertop. She has treated her sensitivities with injections, multiple vitamins and ionizers, cotton blankets and pillows, bottled water, oxygen tanks, aluminum foil.

In 1987, after following a macrobiotic diet for six months, she experienced major improvement. The excruciating shoulder pain disappeared, and over the next few months every chronic symptom that she ever had vanished. During the next few years, she gave up her allergy injections and could remain up to fourteen hours a day in a toxic, smoke-filled environment.

"In three years she'll be fifty, yet she's stronger and healthier now than she has ever been in her life," concluded a profile in *The Human Ecologist*. "She takes no medications, no supplements, no injections, and for the first time in her life, has no symptoms."

Source: Sherry A. Rogers, M.D., "From HEAL's Advisory Board: The Cure Is in the Kitchen — One Case History," *The Human Ecologist*, Fall, 1990, pp. 19-21.

124. Lupus

In laboratory studies, a low-calorie, low-fat diet benefited mice with lupus, an autoimmune disorder that affects the connective tissue. A researcher at the University of Florida theorized that limiting animal fat and protein, especially from beef, pork, lamb, and dairy food, would have similar effects in humans.

Source: L. C. Corman, "The Role of Diet in Animal Models of Systemic Lupus Erythematosus: Possible Implications for Human Lupus," *Seminars in Arthritis and Rheumatism*15:61-69, 1985.

125. Candida Albicans

Candida albicans is a fungal microorganism that exists naturally in the linings of the digestive, respiratory, and reproductive organs in low concentrations. However, high concentrations can cause a variety of symptoms including fatigue, depression, food allergies, chemical sensitivity, and other symptoms. "Candida" — the popular name for this yeast-related illness (YRI) — has been associated with immune deficiency, and researchers have linked it with excessive use of antibiotics, oral contraceptives, treatment with corticosteroids, and a diet high in sugar and simple carbohydrates.

In a review of candida, Elmer Cranton, M.D., a former president of the American Holistic Medical Association, recommended dietary treatment including avoidance of simple sugars that promote the growth of yeast, soft drinks, and alcohol. He also recommended temporary minimization of breads and baked goods and some cereals which may trigger symptoms as part of the healing response. "As improvement occurs, intake of complex carbohydrate [rice, oats, barley, etc.] may be increased to a more desirable level," he emphasized.

Source: E. M. Cranton, "Candida Albicans: A Common Cause of Fatigue and Depression," *Journal of Holistic Medicine* 8:3-14, 1986.

8

Benefits for Mother and Child

In his writings on the embryo, Leonardo da Vinci observed, "The mother desires a certain food and the child bears the mark of it." The importance of prenatal and postnatal nutrition has become better known in recent years. Breastfeeding has received overwhelming scientific and medical support after decades of being out of fashion. In the field of pediatrics, cardiologists are now identifying heart disease as a disease that begins with improper diet in infancy and childhood and progresses through young adulthood and middle age. The discovery that Vitamin B_{12} is available in miso, tempeh, seaweed, and other plant-quality foods has also helped popularize a low-fat, high-fiber diet for mother and child.

126. Vegetarian and Macrobiotic Children

• In a study of vegetarian preschool children, researchers at New England Medical Center Hospital in Boston found that the growth of macrobiotic youngsters did not significantly differ from those of non-macrobiotics before age two. After age two, macrobiotic children tended to put on weight more quickly than the children brought up on yoga diets, Seventh-Day Adventist diets, or other vegetarian regimes. Nearly all the children had been breastfed, and it was found that macrobiotic children who had been weaned did not differ in caloric intake from nonmacrobiotics.

Source: M.W. Shull et al., "Velocities of Growth in Vegetarian Preschool Children," *Pediatrics* 60:410-17, 1977.

• In a study of 119 vegetarian and macrobiotic children with a mean age of about two years, Boston nutritionists reported they were generally smaller, leaner, and lighter than nonvegetarian children. Despite varying degrees of avoidance of meat and other animal foods, consumption of protein, carbohydrate, and fat in the diets of those children age one year or older who were no longer being breastfed fell within normal levels.

Source: J. T. Dwyer et al., "Preschoolers on Alternate Life-Style Diets," *Journal of the American Dietetic Association* 72:264-70, 1978.

IQs of Vegetarian and Macrobiotic Children					
Type of Vegetarian Diet	Number	Chronological Age Mean	Chronological Age Range	Mean Mental Age	Mean IQ
macrobiotic		months	months	months	points
vegan	6	50.0	35-69	66.5	119.3
vegetarian	11	56.1	25-100	66.9	111.3
total	17	53.9	25-100	65.8	114.1
other	11	41.7	24-83	53.6	118.3
total -- all subjects	28	49.1	24-100	61.6	115.8
Source: Journal of the American Dietetic Association, 1980					

127. Diet and I.Q.

In a study of mental development and I.Q., macrobiotic and vegetarian children were significantly brighter and more intelligent than ordinary youngsters their age. The test group consisted of twenty-eight children in the Boston area between two and eight years old, with a mean age of four years old. The mean I.Q. was 116 for the group as a whole, or 16 percent above average. The children's mean mental age was found to exceed their mean chronologic age by approximately a year. The macrobiotic children's I.Q.'s and mental ages were slightly higher than the other vegetarians. "In the judgments of both the pediatrician and psychologic technician, the children as a group were bright," the researchers concluded. They speculated, however, that the brightness may be due to better education on the part of the macrobiotic and vegetarian parents, not to diet.

Source: J. T. Dwyer et al., "Mental Age and I.Q. of Predominantly Vegetarian Children," *Journal of the American Dietetic Asociation* 76:142-47, 1980.

128. Breastfeeding and Cancer

• Breast-feeding can reduce the risk of certain cancers for both mother and child. Researchers from the National Institute of Child Health and Human Development in Bethesda, MD., found that infants breast-fed more than 6 months had a lower risk of developing cancer in childhood, especially lymphomas.

In this study, children who were formula-fed or breast-fed for less than six months had approximately twice the risk of getting some childhood cancers by age fifteen as those breast-fed for longer than 6 months. They also had five times the risk of getting lymphoma.

"Mother's milk contains substantial antimicrobial benefits for infants, increasing their resistance to many infections and possibly protecting them from many diseases, including lymphomas," researchers reported.

Source: "Breast-Feeding Linked to Decreased Cancer Risk for Mother, Child," *Journal of the National Cancer Institute* 80:1362-63, 1988.

• In a Chinese medical study, researchers found that the longer the mother nursed, the less at risk she was of breast cancer. Mimi Yu, Associate Professor of Preventive Medicine at the University of Southern California in Los Angeles, studied more than 500 Chinese women with breast cancer in Shanghai and 500 healthy women.

The women she studied on an average nursed their various children for a cumulative total of nine years, a common pattern in China. "We believe that long periods of nursing would have the same protective effect for American women," Yu reported.

Source: "Breast-Feeding Linked to Decreased Cancer Risk for Mother, Child," *Journal of the National Cancer Institute* 80:1362-63, 1988.

• An analysis of seventeen pesticides, toxins, and other chemical substances in the breast milk of vegetarian and nonvegetarian mothers found that except for polychlorinated biphenyls (which were about equal) "the highest vegetarian value was lower than the lowest value obtained in the [nonvegetarian] sample. . . [T]he mean vegetarian levels were only one or two percent as high as the average levels in the United States."

Source: J. Hergenrather et al., "Pollutants in Breast Milk of Vegetarians," [Letter], *New England Journal of Medicine* 304:792, 1976.

129. Dairy and Colic

Antibodies in cow milk are the likely cause of colic in babies, and mothers who consume dairy products can pass them on in their breast milk. In a study at Washington University, mothers with colicky babies had significantly higher levels of cow antibodies in their milk as mothers of babies without colic. Colic, characterized by crying spells that can last 3 hours or more, affects about 20 percent of all babies in modern society. Dr. Frank Harris, a spokesman for the American Academy of Pediatrics, said the study told frustrated mothers: "It may not be what you're doing. It may be what you're eating."

Source: "Cow Antibodies Are Linked to Colic in Babies," *New York Times*, March 30, 1991 and *Pediatrics*, April, 1991.

130. Children and Heart Disease

• Top American health officials joined in calling for a low-fat, low-cholesterol diet for everyone over age two to prevent heart disease in later life, not just for adults at risk for heart attacks and other cardiovascular disease. The recommendations, sponsored by a panel convened by the National Heart, Lung and Blood Institute and the Cholesterol Education Program and endorsed by a coalition of forty-two major health and medical organizations, called for the cholesterol testing of all children whose parents or grandparents had heart attacks or other cardiovascular problems, including a parent with blood cholesterol over 240.

The panel called for reductions in fat consumption and for intake of more grains, vegetables, and fruit.

Groups that endorsed the report included the American Medical Association, the American College of Physicians, the American Public Health Association, the U.S. Food and Drug Administration,

Cholesterol and Diet in Boys Aged 7 to 9			
	Saturated fat (% of total calories eaten)	Dietary cholesterol (mg/1,000 calories)	Blood cholesterol count (mg/dl)
Ghana	10.5	48	128
Philippines	9.3	97	147
Italy	10.4	159	159
U.S.	13.5	151	167
Netherlands	15.1	142	174
Finland	17.7	157	190
Source: National Center for Health Statistics, 1991			

the U.S. Department of Agriculture, and the U.S. Department of Health and Human Services.

Source: Warren E. Leary, "Cholesterol Tests Are Recommended for a Quarter of Children," *New York Times,* April 9, 1991.

• In Bogalusa, a semirural Louisiana community, investigators have been monitoring blood values and dietary intake among schoolchildren for a number of years. In 1988, they reported that children had an average cholesterol level 300 mg. and ate a daily diet consisting of an average of 38 percent fat.

Children should be routinely checked for signs of heart disease beginning at age five, proposed Dr. Gerald Berenson, chief cardiologist at the Lousiana State University Medical Center in New Orleans. At an American Heart Association forum in January, 1990, he reported the results of a twenty-five-year study of more than 10,000 children showing that doctors can identify at six months those children who are likely to develop excessively high levels of blood cholesterol. He recommended that children at risk of heart disease should be taught as soon as they begin school to avoid fats in their diet, exercise, keep their weight down, and not smoke cigarettes.

Sources: G. S. Berenson et al., "Cardiovascular Risk Factors in Children and Early Prevention of Heart Disease," *Clinical Chemistry* 34:B115-22, 1988.

131. Vitamin B₁₂ and Diet

Until recently scientists believed that only meat, poultry, fish and other animal quality foods contained Vitamin B_{12}. However, recent studies have shown that tempeh, miso, and other fermented soy products contain B_{12}, as do various sea vegetables. Nursing mothers are especially susceptible to low levels of Vitamin B_{12} because of the demands of their growing baby. Doctors have been concerned about this problem in vegetarian and macrobiotic mothers who eat little or no animal food.

• In 1977 researchers found that the Vitamin B_{12} content of typical samples of tempeh sold commercially in North America ranged from 1.5 to 6.3 micrograms per average 3.5 ounce serving. The adult RDA for B_{12} is 3 micrograms, so the tempeh contained 50 to 210 percent of the recommended daily allowance. Further testing showed that using the bacterium *Klebsiella* in the starter used to make tempeh could raise the B_{12} levels as high as 14.8 micrograms, at which level a 1-ounce serving would supply the RDA.

Source: I. T. H. Liem et al, "Production of Vitamin B_{12} in Tempeh, a Fermented Soybean Food," *Applied and Environmental Microbiology* 34:773-76, 1977.

• A study of macrobiotic and vegetarian mothers suggested that nursing mothers with low Vitamin B_{12} levels could get an acceptable source of this nutrient by consuming sea vegetables that are naturally high in B_{12}. "The relatively high vitamin B_{12} content of sea vegetables is thought to reflect a high content of vitamin B_{12} producing microorganism[s] in these plants. Although these analyses need to be confirmed with further studies, sea vegetables may represent a potentially important source of this vitamin in the strict vegetarian diet."

Source: B. L. Specker et al., "Increased Urinary Methylmalonic Acid Excretion in Breast-Fed Infants of Vegetarian Mothers and Identification of an Acceptable Dietary Source of Vitamin B_{12}," *American Journal of Clinical Nutrition* 47:89-92, 1988.

• In a study of thirty-six men and women in Israel who were not eating animal food, researchers found that B_{12} levels were normal and none of the subjects had any hematologic evidence of deficiency, though four had neurologic complaints. Red blood cell folate levels, complete blood count, including hemoglobin and mean corpuscular volume, were similar in subjects and controls.

The thirty-six subjects had been following their way of eating from five to thirty-five years and participated in various vegetarian communities and study groups. Eleven subjects had not been eating animal food for twenty years or more.

The researchers speculated that sources of B_{12} in their diet could come from microorganisms in legumes, from sea algae, and from "the possibility of intestinal absorption of vitamin B_{12} that is synthesized in the gut."

Sources: P. Bar-Sella, Y. Rakover, and D. Ratner, "Vitamin B_{12} and Folate Levels in Long-Term Vegans," *Israeli Journal of Medical Science* 26:309-12, 1990.

• Animal foods commonly believed to be high in B_{12} may actually be low or deficient. In lab tests commissioned by independent researcher Sylvia Ruth Gray in 1989 and 1990, no identifiable B_{12} was found in beef liver, Swiss cheese, and chicken breast and only 2.19 mcg in beef heart. In the 1960s, similar tests showed these foods contained 122, 1.71, .5, and 14.2 mcg respectively. In contrast, macrobiotic/vegetarian foods measured higher than the animal foods. Sea vegetables measured up to 9 mcg, tempeh to 4 mcg, and miso to .7. Gray attributed the sharp decline in B_{12} levels to environmental pollution and modern chemical agriculture, especially the depletion of cobalt in soils which promotes B_{12} synthesis.

Source: Nathaniel Mead, "Where's the B_{12}?", *Solstice* 39:10-15, 1990; "Here's the B_{12}," *Solstice* 40:10-13, 1990; "Corrections on Vitamin B_{12}," *Solstice* 42:5-7, 1990; Sylvia Ruth Gray, "B_{12} Update," *Solstice* 43:5-7, 1990; Sylvia Ruth Gray, "B_{12} Update," *Solstice* 44:6-8, 1990. For further information and to support further research, contact Sylvia Ruth Gray, 315 First Ave., Salt Lake City, UT 84103.

132. Soyfoods for Children

In 1983 the U.S.D.A. approved the use of soy products and other vegetable protein products as partial substitutes for meats, poultry, and seafoods in school lunch and some other feeding programs. In a review of the health benefits of soy, researchers from the Department of Food Science at the University of Illinois noted:

• Soy products were comparable with milk in protein quality for preschool and older children.

• Except for premature infants, soy protein can serve as a sole protein source in the human diet.

• Soyfoods are high in protease inhibitors that inhibit the action of various enzymes that have been associated with causing cancer.

• Soy formulas are lactose free and may benefit infants and small children who are sensitive to cow-milk protein which can cause diarrhea, emesis, vomiting, and weight loss.

• Soy products can reduce cholesterol and triglycerides in subjects with high lipid levels and protect against heart disease.

• Soy foods are useful in decreasing blood glucose responses compared with other high-fiber foods and may prevent diabetes.

"One desirable way to alter typical American diet patterns to meet the above [National Academy of Science, WHO, USDA] dietary recommendations involves partial replacement of foods of animal origin with cereals and legumes...

"Although at the present time soy protein makes up only a small component of the American diet, it is expected that the many positive aspects of soy will result in increasingly greater human use of this legume. A whole variety of low-cost, highly functional soy-protein products are available for use."

Source: John W. Erdman, Jr. and Elizabeth J. Fordyce, "Soy Products and the Human Diet," *American Journal of Clinical Nutrition* 49:725-37, 1989.

• In tests of the acceptability of tofu in the lunch menus of preschoolers, analysis showed that the nutritional quality of the nine tofu recipes adhered more closely to dietary guidelines than the beef, chicken, eggs, and cheese originally served. The children accepted the tofu well, preferring it to dairy and meat in several dishes including macaroni and cheese, lasagna, tuna casserole, and quiche.

Source: H. L. Ashraf et al., , "Use of Tofu in Preschool Meals," *Journal of the American Dietetic Association* 90:114-16, 1990.

133. Vegetables and Malnutrition

Orange and yellow vegetables high in vitamin A could help save the lives of millions of malnourished children. In a study of 15,000 underfed preschool children in India, researchers found that those given dietary supplements were twice as likely to live as those who did not receive the vitamin A. As in many developing countries, those who died did so largely from chronic diarrhea.

Source: L. Rahmathullah et al., "Reduced Mortality Among Children in South India Receiving a Small Weekly Dose of Vitamin A," *New England Journal of Medicine* 323:929-35, 1990.

9

Keeping Fit, Enhancing Sexuality & Prolonging Life

Complex carbohydrates from whole grains, vegetables, seaweed, fruit, and other plant-quality food enter the digestive system gradually, supplying the body with an even, steady source of energy. In contrast, meat and sugar, and other high-caloric foods, provide an initial burst of power but quickly fade. Scientific and medical studies, as well as practical results on the playing field, in the home and office, and during times of war and scarcity, are confirming that people eating a diet centered on grains and vegetables have more strength, endurance, and vitality and live longer than people eating the modern diet.

134. Food and Endurance

• In New Haven, Connecticut, Irving Fisher devised tests to measure diet and endurance of Yale athletes eating animal food, vegetarian athletes (from the Battle Creek Sanitarium in Michigan), and vegetarians who were sedentary. The tests included holding the arms outstretched as long as possible, deep knee bends until exhaustion, and repeated leg raises. The vegetarians excelled in all three tests, and the sedentary vegetarians generally exhibited stronger endurance than the athletic meat-eaters.

"The results of the comparisons . . . would indicate that the us-

Diet, Exercise, and Endurance						
	Arm Holding		Deep Knee Bending		Leg Raising	
Type of Diet and Exercise	Number	Average	Number	Average	Number	Average
Meat-Eating Athletes	15	10 minutes	9	383 times	6	279 times
Vegetarian Athletes	19	39 minutes	16	927 times	6	288 times
Sedentary Athletes	13	64 minutes	5	535 times	1	74 times

Source: Yale Medical Journal, 1907

ers of [low-protein] and the non-flesh dietaries have far greater endurance than those who are accustomed to the ordinary American diet," Fisher concluded.

Source: Irving Fisher, "The Influence of Flesh Eating on Endurance," *Yale Medical Journal* 13:205-21, 1907.

• In tests with stationary bicycle to measure energy output, Danish researchers put nine men on a mixed meat and vegetable diet. After three days, the average time pedaled was 1 hour and 54 minutes. On a high-protein diet rich in milk, meat, and eggs, the average time pedaled after three days was 57 minutes. When put on a diet of whole grain cereals, bread, vegetables, and fruit, their mean endurance increased to 2 hours 47 minutes.

Source: Per-Olf Astrand, "Somthing Old and Something New . . . Very New," *Nutrition Today* 3:(2) 9-11, 1968.

135. Macrobiotic Baseball Team

In 1983 a Japanese professional baseball team climbed from last place to first place by switching to a macrobiotic diet. After taking over the last place Seibu Lions in October, 1981, manager Tatsuro Hirooka initiated a dietary experiment. Restricting the players' intake of meat, sugar, and white rice, he instructed them to eat brown rice, tofu, vegetables, and soybean products. He told the men that animal food increases an athlete's susceptibility to injuries. Conversely, natural foods, they were told, protect the body from sprains and dislocations and keep the mind clear and focused. During the 1982 season, the Lions were ridiculed by their archrivals, the Nippon Ham-Fighters, a team sponsored by a major meat company. However, the Lions defeated the Ham-Fighters for the Pacific League crown and continued to the Japan World Series and beat the Chunichi Dragons. The Lions won the championship again the following year as well.

Source: "The Veggie Baseball Team," *Parade Magazine,* April 15, 1984.

136. Diet and Impotence

Atherosclerosis has been implicated in a majority of impotence in American men. This condition, which affects about 10 million American men, including 25 percent over the age of 65, is brought on by hardening of the arteries caused by too much fat in the diet.

In a study of 440 impotent men, researchers found evidence of arterial lesion in the penises of 53 percent. "Our results indicate that much of the increase in impotence with age is associated with arteriosclerotic changes in the arteries and cavernous tissue," the investigators concluded. "Impotent patients should follow the regimens [diets] recommended to patients with more severe arteriosclerosis of other sites."

Source: R. Virag, P. Bouilly, and D. Frydman, "Is Impotence an Arterial Disorder?" *Lancet* I:181-84, 1985.

137. Diet and Sexual Vitality

After counseling thousands of people, macrobiotic educator Michio Kushi concluded that diet has a profound influence on sexuality. "Female sexuality depends upon the smooth flow of upward, yin energy in the body. At the moment of orgasm, sensations orginating in the vagina and clitoris radiate up through the pelvis and along the primary channel to the upper chakras [energy centers]. Animal foods are strongly charged with the opposite or downward (yang) energy, and when eaten in excess inhibit the natural unfolding of upward energy in the female body. Animal foods tighten and constrict the chakras and can limit the range of pleasure and depth of emotion that a woman experiences during sex. . . . This is a leading cause of the inability to achieve orgasm during intercourse."

In women, he observed, animal food consumption is also connected with fibroid tumors, blockages in the Fallopian tubes, dermoid cysts, vaginal discharge, and in extreme cases cancer of the ovaries, uterus, or cervix — conditions which can interfere with healthy sexuality.

In men, excessive animal food intake can lead to prostate enlargement, premature ejaculation, or exclusive "concentration on orgasm without the more total involvement of the mind and emotions." Meanwhile, sugar, dairy food, tropical fruits, and other more expansive (yin) food can diminish sexual vitality and lead to impotence.

"The complex carbohydrates in whole grains, beans, and fresh local vegetables have a number of advantages in helping to promote sexual harmony," Kushi reported. "Because they are slowly broken down and absorbed into the bloodstream, they provide a slow, steady supply of energy. This contributes to endurance and staying power." In particular, he recommended brown rice, miso soup, root vegetables such as burdock, carrot, and jinenjo (Japanese mountain potato), beans (especially adzuki beans), sea vegetables, and gomashio (sesame seed salt) to enhance sexual potency.

Source: Michio Kushi with Edward and Wendy Esko, *The Gentle Art of Making Love* (Garden City Park, N.Y.: Avery Publishing, 1990).

138. White Flour and Short Life

In the early 19th century, in feeding trials with animals, M. Magendie, a French scientist, found that refined flour was unable to support life. "A dog fed on fine white bread and water, both at discretion, does not live beyond the fiftieth day. . . . A dog fed on the coarse [barley] bread of the military, lives and keeps his health."

Source: C. Londe, "On Aliment," *Lancet* 10:829-35, 1826.

139. Caloric-Restricted Diets

• Caloric restriction without vitamin or mineral deficiency can extend life, retard some disease, and possibly even slow the aging process, according to a joint study by the Food and Drug Administration and the National Institute on Aging. In the study involving twenty-four laboratories, half of the rats and mice were given unlimited access to food and the other half were restricted to about 60 percent of the calories. About 80 percent of the calorie-restricted mice were alive after 28 months, compared to just 50 percent of the others, reported Ronald Hart, director of the FDA's National Center for Toxicological Research in Jefferson, Arkansas.

None of the calorie-restricted rodents had cancer after 30 months, while 25 percent of the controls had malignant tumors. "These animals are living longer, healthier, more active lives," said Hart.

Source: "Hungry Rats Live Longer," *Boston Globe*, Dec. 5, 1988.

• In longevity experiments, scientists reported that mice fed a calorie-restricted diet lived an average of 55 months compared to 36 months for rodents allowed to eat as much as they wished.

"The outcome of calorie restriction is spectacular," said Richard Weindruch, a gerontologist at the National Institute on Aging in Bethesda, Md. "Gerontologists have tried many things to extend life span, but this is the only one that consistently works in the lab."

Experiments showed that the restricted diet prevented heart disease, diabetes, and kidney failure, retarded all types of cancer, eliminated or forestalled cataracts, gray hair, and feebleness, protected the genes against environmental insult, kept important enzymes operating at peak efficiency, and cut back on dangerous metabolic byproducts in the body.

Rats on restricted diets, for example, almost never came down with kidney or heart disease, kept their shiny white coats, were able to run mazes more successfully than the well-fed rats, and had immune systems that remained strong well into old age. They lived to nearly 50 months and died of natural causes. "Right now, the maximum human life span is about 110 years, and only a few people live to that age," said Dr. Roy L. Walford of U.C.L.A., a pioneer in calorie-restricted diets. "But if what is true for other species is true for man, then with a sufficiently vigorous caloric restriction, the maximum life span could be extended to about 170."

Dr. Walford himself follows a low-calorie diet of about 1,500 to 2,000 calories a day, compared with an average daily intake of 2,500 calories for men (and 2,100 for women). The majority of his calories come from grains, vegetables, and other natural foods.

Source: Natalie Angier, "Diet Offers Tantalizing Clues to Long Life," *New York Times*, Science Section, April 17, 1990.

Effect of Food Restriction During War on Mortality in Copenhagen, Denmark			
Year	Deaths from All Diseases*	Deaths from Epidemic Diseases & TB	Deaths from Other Diseases	Ratio (Average = 100)
1907	145	31	114	105
1908	152	35	117	107
1909	142	31	111	102
1910	135	26	109	100
1911	148	32	116	106
1912	138	30	108	99
1913	130	28	102	94
1914	133	27	106	97
1915	134	26	106	97
1916	145	35	110	101
1917	123	33	90	83
1918**	99	27	72	66

*Number of deaths per ten thousand men between the ages 25 and 65

**From Oct. 1, 1917 to Oct. 1, 1918

Source: *Journal of the American Medical Association, 1920*

140. Diet and World War I

During World War I, Mikkel Hindhede, M.D., Superintendent of the State Institute of Food Research, persuaded the Danish government to shift its agricultural priorities from raising grain for livestock to grain for direct human consumption. Accordingly, in the face of a foreign blockade, the Danes ate primarily barley, whole-rye bread, green vegetables, potatoes, milk, and some butter. In the nation's capital, the death rate from all causes, including cancer, fell 34 percent during 1917 to 1918. "It was a low protein experiment on a large scale, about 3 million subjects being available," Hindhede reported to his medical colleagues. " . . . People entered no complaints; there were no digestive troubles, but we are accustomed to the use of whole bread and we knew how to make such bread of good quality."

Source: M. Hindhede, "The Effects of Food Restriction During War on Mortality in Copenhagen," *Journal of the American Medical Association* 74:381-82, 1920.

141. Diet and World War II

During World War II, rates of cancer, heart disease, and other degenerative illnesses declined as a result of wartime restrictions on articles in the modern diet. For example, in England and Wales, breast cancer mortality markedly fell as consumption of sugar, meat, and fat declined and consumption of grains and vegetables increased. By 1954, fat consumption returned to prewar levels, and breast cancer levels subsequently climbed to previous levels.

Source: D. M. Ingram, "Trends in Diet and Breast Cancer Mortality in England and Wales, 1928-1977," *Nutrition and Cancer* 3(2):75-80, 1982.

142. Diet and the Vietnam War

• In April 1965, Professors Suzuki and Sakaida from Japan were captured by Vietnamese revolutionaries. At first they thought they would become malnourished or ill on their meager diet, but as their captivity continued they discovered just the opposite.

"The Vietcong fed us rice and a soup made from wild cassava leaves, every day, three times a day. . . At first we were very worried about such a meagre diet. But to our astonishment, none of us ever got ill or tired, despite having to walk twenty or thirty miles a day through thick virgin jungle. . . It's very odd, but we never got sick with that freshly hulled rice! No sign of malaria either!"

Source: George Ohsawa, *The Macrobiotic*, #108, pp. 4-5.

• In 1977 a study of seventy-eight former U.S. Navy prisoners of war in Vietnam showed that they had less endocrine, nutritional, and metabolic diseases, as well as less circulatory, nervous system, genito-urinary, and musculoskeletal diseases, than other Navy pilots. The researchers cited the Vietnamese diet — high in rice and vegetables and low in dietary cholesterol and fat — as a major factor in their better physical health. "In contrast to the life of the POWs during confinement, control group members usually had access to an abundant diet — high in animal fat — to tobacco, to alcohol, and experienced the stresses of their jobs where only excellent performance was rewarded by promotions."

Source: John A. Plag, Ph.D., "American POWS from Vietnam: Follow-Up Studies of the Subsequent Health and Adjustment of the Men and Their Families" (San Diego: Naval Health Research Center, 1977).

10

A Calm, Peaceful Mind

"Of all the areas of promising nutrition research and knowledge, the relationship between nutrition and mental health and development is the least funded and probably the least well understood," George McGovern noted during the Dietary Goals hearings in 1977. "Established scientific thinking remains weighted against those few scientists and practitioners who are striving to understand the complex links between the food we consume and how we think and behave as individuals. According to the National Institute of Mental Health, 6.4 million Americans are under some form of mental health care and an estimated 10 percent of all Americans are in need of such care. That translates into over 20 million people, and if further research is undertaken along a nutritonal line we could find that a significant number of mental health problems could be cured or prevented by better nutrition." According to the Institute of Medicine, in 1989 7.5 million children in the United States, representing 12 percent of the population under eighteen, suffered from a mental disorder or emotional disturbance, and few were receiving treatment.

143. Food and the Brain

At Massachusetts Institute of Technology (MIT), researchers have investigated the effects of food on the brain and nervous system. "It is becoming increasingly clear that brain chemistry and function can be influenced by a single meal. That is, in well-nourished individuals consuming normal amounts of food, short-term changes in food composition can rapidly affect brain function," explained Dr. John Fernstrom.

According to scientists, whole grains and other foods high in complex carbohydrates have the capacity to increase the brain's intake of tryptophan, an amino acid that aids in relief of pain and in lowering blood pressure. Tryptophan has also been associated in studies with lifting depression and improving sleep. In contrast to grains and vegetables, meals high in animal protein lower levels of tryptophan reaching the brain. This "growing body of information now points to new clinically useful applications of tryptophan and thus also for the use of specific meals that would increase tryptophan levels," Fernstrom concluded.

Source: Tom Monte, "A Nutritional Approach to Mental Health," Michio Kushi et al., *Crime and Diet* (Tokyo & New York: Japan Publications, 1987), pp. 146-47.

144. Food and Psychiatry

In addition to tryptophan which comes from protein but requires carbohydrates to enter the brain and can lift depression and cause sleepiness, psychiatrists are looking at the role of other dietary factors such as tyrosine (an ingredient in animal protein which buffers effects of stress) and choline (from soy lecithin that can shorten manic attacks). "It seemed absurd to psychiatrists that what you eat could directly influence the brain," said Dr. van Praag, in a recent issue of *Integrative Psychiatry*. "By now, though, the data from animals and people is hard to deny. The question is how far we can go in finding useful applications in psychiatry."

Source: Daniel Goleman, "Food and Brain: Psychiatrists Explore Use of Nutrients in Treating Disorders," *New York Times*, Science Section, March 1, 1988.

145. Hypoglycemia and Mental Illness

A sampling of 300 psychiatric patients found that about 40 percent were hypoglycemic, a condition characterized by low blood sugar levels brought on by excessive consumption of sugar and other simple carbohydrates. Another study found a 70 percent rate of chronic hypoglycemia in diagnosed schizophrenics. In a group of 220 patients with neuroses with primary complaint of anxiety or depression, 205 were determined to be hypoglycemic. Further studies with 700 patients found 90 percent hypoglycemic. When treated for this blood glucose problem only, the psychiatric problems began to clear up within ten days in the majority of patients.

Sources: H. M. Saltzer, M.D., "Relative Hypoglycemia as a Cause of Neuropsychiatric Illness," *Journal of the National Medical Association* 58:12-19, p. 27 and E. M. Abrahamson, M.D. and A. Pezet, *Body, Mind and Sugar* (New York: Avon Books, 1977), p. 109.

146. Diet and Psychiatry

Dr. Stephen Harnish, a New Hampshire psychiatrist, reported that macrobiotics had benefited many of his patients who were chronically and severely mentally ill. Citing several case histories, he described a young woman with a history of severe depression who had been in a state hospital for two years and treated with antidepressants and antipsychotic medications. Tests by Dr. Harnish's department found that the woman was hypoglycemic and administration of a macrobiotic diet high in complex carbohydrates and one that avoided animal food and sugar resulted in steady improvement, reduced medication, and return to normal functioning. "She now has motivation to do new things and has made plans to return to school." Another patient, a middle-aged woman diagosed with manic depressive illness and told she would be on medication the rest of her life, learned to recognize her moods swings on a macrobiotic diet, was weaned of medication, and is now functional.

Noting that hundreds of other psychiatric patients could benefit from this approach, Dr. Harnish concluded, "One possible way to do this could be to set up and staff group homes for the mentally ill with macrobiotic staff (cooks and counselors) which are associated with psychiatric care providers who are sensitive to the patients' dietary needs and who will document data on the condition of these patients as they change their diets and lives."

Source: Stephen Harnish, M.D., "On My Awakening to the Macrobiotic Way," in Edward Esko, editor, *Doctors Look at Macrobiotics* (Tokyo & New York: Japan Publications, 1988), pp. 151-68.

147. Mental Health in Africa

In 1971, a South African doctor observed, "Regarding mental disease in the people of the Transkei, I can say that in the past eleven years I have not diagnosed a single case of schizophrenia in a tribal African living on an unrefined carbohydrate diet, whereas this disease is the commonest psychosis among the urbanized Africans."

Dr. G. Daynes attributed the development of mental illness to white sugar and refined corn flour.

Source: T. L. Cleave, *The Saccharine Disease* (Bristol: John Wright & Sons), 1974, p. 25.

148. Macrobiotics and Schizophrenia

With the help of his mother, Charlotte Mahoney-Briscoe, David Briscoe healed himself of schizophrenia by adhering to a balanced macrobiotic diet. David, diagnosed with mental and emotional illness in the 1960s, unsuccessfully tried many hospitals, medications, and confinement before changing his diet. "He might as well be dead," his mother said looking back. David developed an exaggerated appetite for sugar: candy, cookies, and ice cream, as well as steak, very salty foods like crackers and potato chips, and diet soda. In high school, he become physically ill, with acute kidney problems, frequent sore throats, digestive problems, fevers, and a duodenal ulcer. For his depression, he went to psychiatrists for six years and became addicted to Thorazine. After changing his way of eating to brown rice, tamari soy sauce, and other foods, he made a complete recovery. David is currently married, the father of four children, and director of the Macrobiotic Center of Kansas City.

Source: David Briscoe and Charlotte Mahoney-Briscoe: *A Personal Peace: Macrobiotic Reflections on Mental and Emotional Recovery* (Tokyo and New York: Japan Publications, 1989).

11

A Safe, Harmonious Community

From the individual, health radiates to the home, the school, the work-place, and the community as a whole. At the social level, current scientific and medical studies are associating the modern way of eating — especially sugar and other highly processed foods — with hyperactivity and learning disabilities, crime and antisocial activity, and other imbalanced behavior. Meanwhile, vegetarian and macrobiotic dietary changes have been success-fully implemented in a number of schools, hospitals, and prisons.

149. Diet and Hyperactivity

Hyperactivity, learning disabilities, and allergic reactions are epidemic in modern schools and have been associated with chemi-cals, artificial food colors and flavorings, and highly processed foods. In the U.S., estimates of hyperactivity in schoolchildren range from one in three to one in twenty, while in England and other countries where food colors are regulated, only one in 2000 is re-ported hyperactive.

Source: D. Divoky, "Toward a Nation of Sedated Children," *Learning*, March 1973, pp. 6-13.

150. Diet and Biosocial Decline

In testimony before the Senate Select Committee on Nutrition and Human Needs, Dr. Carolyn Brown, director of a school for learning disabled children in Berkeley, California, pointed to the social effects of changes in diet and lifestyle since World War II:

"Let us look for a moment at a few interesting health and social statistics. The members of this committee know well the evidence of the increase in synthetic foods, and other nutritional changes. . . . What do we know about what has happened to the children that grew up during these twenty-five years? We know that there was a sixfold increase in arrests of children under fifteen suspected of murder, non-negligent manslaughter, aggravated assault, and rape. The factor increase was three for fifteen to seventeen year olds, two for eighteen to twenty-five year olds. We know that 'accidents' resulting in death rose dramatically among the young, that divorce rates have continued to increase, that suicides have been rising among young people in comparison to the rest of the population. And we know that there has been an unprecedented fourteen-year decline in the scores of our most gifted children on the Scholastic Aptitude Tests. . . During the eight years from 1958 to 1966, children under seventeen with chronic health problems increased from 18.8 to 24.6 percent. Those from seventeen to twenty-four showed an increase from 39 to 44.4 percent. . . .

"I would like to ask you senators, when we know what has happened during the past twenty-five years in terms of the increase in non-nutritous foods, radiation exposure, television exposure, and exposure to enviromental toxins — and when we know that children born during that period show a dramatic increase in juvenile delinquency, arrest for serious crimes, chronic health problems, and low scores on Scholastic Aptitude Tests — is it not at least a fair question whether we are exposing our children on the whole to an increasingly powerful set of environmental stressors that is producing a broad range of forms of biosocial decline?"

Source: Testimony of Carolyn Brown, Senate Select Committee on Nutrition and Human Needs, 1977.

151. Diet and Learning Disabilities

• In a study of learning disabilities in children, researchers reported that diets high in refined carbohydrates raised cadmium levels, which have been associated with reduced cognitive functioning. Intellectual ability was also negatively correlated with refined food independent of cadmium, age, race, sex, and socioeconomic status.

Source: M.L. Lester et al., "Refined Carbohydrate Intake, Hair Cadmium Levels and Cognitive Functioning in Children," *Journal of Nutrition & Behavior* 1:3-13, 1982.

• When put on a diet centered on whole grains, complex carbohydrates, and unprocessed foods, sixteen children with learning and behavioral problems showed significant improvements in behavior, learning, and intelligence compared to sixteen controls over a twenty-two-week trial period. Further, cadmium and iron levels, which have been linked to learning disabilities, fell 28 and 49 percent respectively.

Source: M. and L. Colgan, "Do Nutrient Supplements and Dietary Changes Affect Learning and Emotional Reactions of Children with Learning Difficulties? A Controlled Series of 16 Cases," *Nutrition and Health* 3:69-77, 1984.

152. Sugar and Aggressive Behavior

Scientists at Yale University have linked sugar consumption by children with abnormal behavior. Research presented in May, 1990, at the annual meeting of the Society for Pediatric Research showed that a concentrated dose of sugar elevated blood levels of adrenaline in children up to ten times higher than normal. Adrenaline, associated with the fight-or-flight response in emergencies, can lead to anxiety, irritability, hyperactivity, or aggression. The scientists said sugar might make the children cranky, anxious, and unfocused.

Source: Jane Brody, "New Data on Sugar and Child Behavior," *New York Times*, May 10, 1990.

153. Macrobiotic Nutritional Studies

* Researchers at the University of Rhode Island studied seventy-six macrobiotic people and reported they generally met currently acceptable medical and nutritional guidelines, including mean values for hemoglobin, hematocrit, serum iron, and transferrin saturation, serum ascorbid acid, vitamin A, beta-carotene, riboflavin, vitamin B_{12}, and folate.

Source: J. G. Bergan and P. T. Brown, "Nutritional Status of 'New' Vegetarians," *Journal of the American Dietetic Association* 76:151-55, 1980.

• In experiments at the University of London, some of the

foods commonly consumed by people on a macrobiotic diet were analysed and the values used to create a data base. The dietary intakes of ten people practicing macrobiotics were assessed by means of a seven-day weighed food record. When the mean daily nutrient intakes were calculated using a computer program and compared to the United Kingdom Recommended Daily Amounts, they were found to be adequate in all of the major nutrients. All of the other nutrients either met the RDA's or, as for vitamins A and C, thiamine, calcium, and iron, "far exceeded the recommendations."

"The macrobiotic diet as eaten by the participants of this study was found to conform with many of the recommendations put forward by recent [medical and scientific] reports on eating for health," according to the chief researcher.

Source: Alison Hinds, BSc., "A Short Study of the Macrobiotic Diet" (London: Queen Elizabeth College, University of London, 1985).

• A Czechoslovakian study of macrobiotic and vegetarian people has found generally healthy nutritional levels. Ludmilla Ruskova, a Prague medical doctor, reported that blood counts and lipid values were excellent compared to the general population. Iron levels, however, were lower, apparently because "it is hard at times to get greens, especially during winter and early spring."

Source: *One Peaceful World*, Autumn/Winter, 1990, p. 3.

155. Natural Foods in a British Nursery School

A British nutritionist found that a macrobiotic day-care center in London not only "supported normal growth" in nursery school children but also could be used as a model to implement national dietary guidelines. Comparing the nutritional adequacy of macrobiotic meals provided preschool children by the Community Health Foundation with ordinary meals at a nursery in Notting Hill, the investigator found that the macrobiotic food consisting of brown rice and other whole grains, miso soup, vegetables, beans, sea vegetables, and other supplemental foods met current U.K.-R.D.I. dietary, energy, and nutrient standards and that the children's anthropometric measurements including weight, height, and skinfold thicknesses were normal.

In contrast, the ordinary nursery school diet was high in dairy food, lard, and other saturated fats that have been associated with the development of atherosclerosis beginning in childhood. "The diet composition of children in Group I [standard nursery] could be made more desirable by a reduction in the amount of full-cream milk and meat and an increase in the amount of cereal foods . . .," the researcher concluded. "The total diet of Group II [macrobiotic nursery] met the U.S. Dietary Goals for fat, sugar, and carbohydrate content, although the home diets of the children were similar to that of the general population. This illustrates the power and potential of nursery meals to contribute to the adoption of a nutritionally sound and beneficial national diet."

Source: Valerie Ventura, "A Comparative Study of the Meals Provided for Pre-School Children by Two Day Nurseries" (London: Department of Nutrition, Queen Elizabeth College, 1980).

155. Tofu Goes to College

When tofu replaced meat, eggs, and dairy food as the main protein source in twelve recipes in a college cafeteria, researchers found that it increased nutrition and was well accepted by the students. The only two recipes found lacking were those for tofu nuggets, which had a poor texture, and tofu chocolate mint pie. In the latter recipe, students disliked not the tofu but the mint flavoring.

Source: H. L. Ashraf and D. Luczycki, "Acceptability of Tofu-Containing Foods among College Students," *Journal of Nutrition Education* 22:137-40, 1990.

156. Macrobiotics in a Boston Hospital

In 1980, a macrobiotic lunch program was started at the Lemuel Shattuck Hospital in Boston for doctors, nurses, and staff. Overall response was favorable and improved noticably after the macrobiotic food line was integrated with the regular cafeteria line. By the second year, half of the food served each day in the cafeteria was prepared macrobiotically. Regular attendance increased from about sixty to 120 to 200 persons each day. At lunch, from 70 to 90 percent of all meals served included at least one item from the macrobiotic menu. "Our surveys documented that the great majority of cafeteria patrons regularly had whole grains, or fresh vegetables, or beans, or dairy-free foods, or sea vegetables, or natural sugar-free deserts, or all of the above in their daily diets," reported Tom Iglehart, consultant to the project, "and for most it was the first such personal innovation in their lifetime. Half of the sheer food *quantity* consumed by the staff from the serving line were macrobiotic dishes."

Dr. William Castelli, director of the Framingham Heart Study, contrasted the healthfulness of the macrobiotic food program at the Shattuck Hospital with ordinary hospital food. "Dr. Robert Wissler, the professor and chairman of the Department of Pathology of the University of Chicago fed the usual house diet of the Billings Hospital [the University of Chicago Medical School's major university hospital] to his baboons and they all lost their legs from atherosclerosis. How our patients are supposed to get well from this is beyond my imagination."

Sources: Tom Iglehart, "The Shattuck Model: Macrobiotics in an Institution," in Michio Kushi et al., *Crime and Diet* (Tokyo and New York: Japan Publications, 1987), pp. 203-29 and William P. Castelli, in Michio Kushi with Tom Igelhart and Eric Zutrau, "Macrobiotics and the American Dream" (Tokyo: Japan Publications, 1986).

157. Whole Foods in an Irish Hospital

Macrobiotic food has been introduced at the National Children's Hospital in Dublin, Ireland. Cecilia Armelin, pediatric dietitian, drew up a sample meal plan including for breakfast: whole oat porridge; for lunch: miso soup with dulse and parsley, brown rice with haricot or adzuki beans, Brussels sprouts, dried apricots and raisins; and for dinner: lentil/barley soup seasoned with miso and parsley and whole grain millet with pears and chopped walnuts. She especially recommended these foods for children with multiple allergies or food intolerance.

Source: Cecilia Armelin, "Wholefood Diet," National Children's Hospital, Dublin, Ireland, 1989.

158. Diet and Geriatric Care

Dr. Jonathan Lieff, Chief of Psychiatry and Geriatric Services at the Shattuck Hospital in Boston and doctors at Tufts University School of Nutrition, designed an experiment in 1982 to test the effect of macrobiotic food on long-term psychiatric and geriatric patients. Some of these people had been confined in the hospital for thirty years or more. In a double-blind study in which neither the ordinary hospital staff or patients knew they were participating, macrobiotic meals avoiding meat, sugar, processed foods, and synthetic food additives and including whole grains, legumes, fresh vegetables and fruits designed to look and taste like regular foods were introduced to a ward of sixteen patients over an eight-week period and eighteen controls. Altogether 187 food items on the macrobiotic menu were prepared, as well as chicken, coffee, and butter which were difficult to simulate. During the test, the researchers noted medically significant reductions in psychosis and agitation among the patients. The scientists found significant improvement in experimental group cooperativeness when compared to the control group, as well as less irritability and improvement upon manifest psychosis. "These data show that the described change in total diet does have a significiantly favorable effect on the health and behavior of geropsychiatric patients," the observers concluded.

Source: Jonathan Lieff et al., "Study Results of Dietary Change in Shattuck Hospital Geropsychiatric Wards, 5 North and 6 North," in Michio Kushi et al., *Crime and Diet* (Tokyo & New York: Japan Publications, 1987), pp. 229-34.

159. Diet in a Brazilian Air Force Academy

The Air Force Academy in Pirasununga, Brazil, 200 kilometers from San Paulo, introduced macrobiotic food in the late 1980s. Almost 600 cadets and officers, including the Academy's deputy commander, joined the "unknown squadron" that volunteered to be served the new food products.

Five cooks from the Academy attended cooking classes at the Macrobiotic Association in Porto Alegro, and after fifteen days' training, returned knowing how to prepare hundreds of dishes with whole grains and vegetables.

The head of the academy's food service, Major Suzeney de Figuiredo Neves predicted, "In three months' time, the volunteers will show good results, and they will be changed into new men."

Source: *Return to Paradise*, Winter 1988-89, p. 3.

160. Diet and Child Abuse

A woman in England with a history of hospitalization for violent behavior and depression and child abuse, including throwing her daughter out of the house through a closed window and knocking her infant son unconscious, was tested for food allergies and found to be suffering from adverse food reactions. After being placed on a restricted diet, she improved, stopped being violent, and went on to get a job and resume normal life in the community.

Source: Richard MacKarness, M.D., *Eating Dangerously* (New York: Harcourt, Brace, Javanovich, 1976).

161. Diet and Stealing

In a double-blind study, Doris J. Rapp, M.D. reported that four young persons with a history of stealing stopped altogether after being place on a restricted diet. However, when the therapy was discontinued and the former diet high in sugar and other refined carbohydrates was resumed, stealing resumed.

Source: Doris J. Rapp, M.D., "Food Allergy Treatment for Hyperkinesis," *Journal of Learning Disabilities* 12(9):42-50, 1979.

162. Diet and Crime

A Cleveland probation official reported a low rate of recidivism among youthful offenders given nutritionally balanced meals. Barbara Reed of the Cuyahoga Falls Muncipal Probation Department reported that of 318 offenders, 252 required attention to their diet, and "we have not had one single person back in court for trouble who has maintained and stayed on the nutritional diet."

Later, Reed reported that more than a thousand ex-offenders had completed her dietary program, and of those who remained on the diet, 89 percent had not been rearrested over the past five years.

Sources: Barbara Reed, statement before the Select Committee on Nutrtion and Human Needs of the U.S. Senate, June 22, 1977 and in Michio Kushi et al., *Crime and Diet* (Tokyo & New York: Japan Publications, 1987), p. 149.

163. Dairy and Crime

Excessive milk consumption is connected with juvenile delinquency in a study by criminologists. Researchers at the University of Washington monitored the dietary intake of thirty chronic youthful offenders and compared them to a group of behaviorally disordered children from the local school district in Tacoma, Washington. They found that the male offenders consumed an average of 64 ounces of milk a day, while the control group rank an average of 30 ounces. For girls, the figures were 35 and 17 ounces respectively. "In some situations," they concluded, "eliminating milk from the diet can result in dramatic improvements in behavior, especially in hyperactive children." They cited other studies showing that up to 90 percent of offenders had a symptom history associated with milk intolerance or allergy.

Source: Alexander Schauss, *Diet, Crime, and Delinquency* (Berkeley, Calif.: Parker House, 1981), pp. 13-14.

164. Sugar and Juvenile Delinquincy

Effect of Sugar on Aggression and Antisocial Behavior in an Incarcerated Juvenile Population		
Frequency of Infractions by Groups	Standard Diet	Sugarless Diet
Low (0 to 1.0 infractions per 10 days)	9 (26%)	11 (46%)
Average (1.1 to 3.0 infractions per 10 days)	13 (38%)	11 (46%)
High (3.1 or more infractions per 10 days)	12 (35%)	2 (8%)
Source: International Journal of Biosocial Research, 1982		

Frank Kern, assistant director at Tidewater Detention Center in Chesapeake, Virginia, a state facility for juvenile offenders, decided to initate some dietary reforms in a macrobiotic direction. In 1979 he arranged an experiment in which sugar was taken out of the meals and snacks of twenty-four inmates. The boys, aged twelve to eighteen, were jailed for offenses that ranged from disorderly conduct, larceny, and burglary to alcohol and narcotics violations. Coke machines were removed from the premises and fruit juice substituted in vending machines for soft drinks, while honey and other milder sweeteners were substituted for refined sugar. The three-month trial was designed as a double-blind case-control study so that neither the detention center personnel nor the inmates knew that they were being tested. At the end of the trial period, the regular staff records on inmates' behavior were checked against a control group of thirty-four youngsters who had been institutionalized previously. Researchers found that the youngsters on the modified diet exhibited a 45 percent lower incidence of formal disciplinary actions and antisocial behavior than the control group. Follow-up studies over the next year showed that after limiting sugar there was an 82 percent reduction in assaults, 77 percent reduction in thefts, 65 percent reduction in horseplay, and 55 percent reduction in refusal to obey orders. The researchers also found that "the people most likely to show improvement were those who had committed violent acts on the outside."

Source: S. Schoenthaler, Ph.D., "The Effect of Sugar on the Treatment and Control of Antisocial Behavior," *International Journal of Biosocial Research* 3(1):1-9, 1982.

165. Macrobiotics in a Portuguese Prison

In 1979 several inmates at the Central Prison in Linho outside of Lisbon, Portugal, began eating macrobiotically and attending lectures on Oriental philosophy and medicine. Soon thirty prisoners had become macrobiotic, and prison officials allowed them to use a large kitchen where they cooked and ate together several times a week. Linho, a maximum security institution, housed Portugal's most dangerous criminals, including José Joaquim (known as "Al Capone"), a celebrated safecracker, and Antonio (To Zé) José Aréal, mastermind of a gang of armed robbers and kidnappers that had been the object of a nation-wide manhunt. As a result of attitude and behavioral changes, To Zé and most of the other prisoners attending classes received commutations and were released early.

"[T]here is a great difference in them, especially in those who have left the prison," Senhor Alfonso, a prison administrator, noted, commenting on the macrobiotic group. "It is not easy to describe — for one thing I can say that now they take more initiative. Actually, there is no problem here with anyone who is macrobiotic; this way of life enjoys a very good reputation. I believe the food and the outside stimulus both helped. The food can change people." To Zé went on to study at the Kushi Institute in Boston and taught macrobiotics in New Bedford, site of a large Portuguese-speaking population, before returning to teach and help other prisoners in Portugal.

Source: Meg Seaker, "Fighting Crime with Diet: Report from a Portuguese Prison," *East West Journal*, July, 1982, pp. 26-34.

12

A Clean, Natural Environment

"The quantity of nutritious vegetable matter consumed in fattening the carcase of an ox," mused Percy B. Shelley, the English poet, in notes to Queen Mab, "would afford ten times the sustenance, undepraving indeed incapable of generating disease, if gathered immediately from the bosom of the earth." In the nearly two centuries since, particularly in the last generation, the effects of the modern way of eating on world health, world hunger, the international economy, and the environment have become more widely appreciated. Alternative agriculture — including organic, sustainable, and natural farming — is the key to returning to a life in harmony with other species and the planet as a whole. Biological transmutation — the controlled, peaceful change of elements into one another — promises in the future to be a healthy, natural alternative to nuclear power, genetic engineering, and other artificial sources of energy and food production.

166. Frances Moore Lappé

In 1971, Frances Moore Lappé compiled information showing that there was enough food to end world hunger but from 50 to 90 percent of the world's grain was fed to livestock rather than people. To get one pound of beef, it takes eighteen pounds of grain and soybeans; pork, six pounds; turkey, four pounds; eggs, three pounds; chicken, three pounds. Meanwhile, pounds of usable protein per acre were tabulated as follows: 356 pounds from soybeans; 260 pounds from rice; 211 pounds from corn; 192 pounds from other legumes; 138 pounds from wheat; 82 pounds from milk; 75 pounds from eggs; 45 pounds from meat of all kinds; and 20 pounds from beef.

Source: Frances Moore Lappé, *Diet for a Small Planet* (New York: Ballantine, 1971).

167. Oil and Food Processing

In 1978, a researcher reported that the modern food and agriculture system uses vast amounts of oil and other fossil fuels. This includes the energy used in the manufacture of heavy farm equipment, chemical fertilizers and pesticides, and in processing and refining. The two major users of energy are the meat and meat products industry and the sugar industry followed by the beverage and soft drink industry. Altogether, per capita use of energy for modern food production and processing comes to the equivalent of 375.4 gallons of oil per year, or about 1 gallon of gasoline a day.

Source: Maurice Green, *Eating Oil: Energy Use in Food Production* (Boulder, Colorado: Westview Press, 1978).

168. U.S.D.A. Organic Agriculture Report

In the early 1980s, the U.S. Department of Agriculture concluded that organic farming can result in substantial energy savings over chemical farming. In a productivity study of organic and inorganic wheat growers in New York and Pennsylvania, the organic farmers used about 30 percent less energy per acre than conventional farmers. However, their yield was 22 percent less, so that the net energy consumption per bushel of organic wheat was about 15 percent less than the wheat grown with chemical fertilizers and pesticides.

Source: U.S. Department of Agriculture, *Report and Recommendations on Organic Farming* (Washington, D.C.: Government Printing Office, 1980).

169. A.A.A.S. Report on Dietary Goals

In 1981 a panel of the American Association for the Advancement of Science met to evaluate the impact of implementing *Dietary Goals for the United States.* Beyond an improvement in public health, the symposium found that dietary changes would have far-reaching social and economic benefits. The scientists concluded that adoption of a diet centered on whole cereal grains rather than meat, poultry, and other animal foods would have significant effects on everything from land, water, fuel, and mineral use to the cost of living, employment rates, and the balance of international trade. Based on government and industry figures, the panel summarized its findings as follows:

Land: production of animal foods uses 85 percent (340/400 million acres) of all cropland, and 95 percent (1,230/1,300 million acres) of all agricultural land in the United States, and it is largely responsible for the extensive abuse of rangeland and forestland and for the loss of soil productivity through erosion and mineral depletion.

Water: production of animal foods uses nearly 80 percent of all piped water in the United States, and it is chiefly responsible for pollution of two-thirds of U.S. basins and for generating over half of the pollution burden entering the nation's lakes and streams.

Wildlife: production of animal foods is responsible for extensive destruction of wildlife through conversion and preemption of forest and rangeland habitats and through massive poisoning and trapping of "predators."

Energy: production, processing, and preparation of animal foods consumes approximately 14 percent of the national energy budget, which is roughly equivalent to the fuel needed to power all our automobiles, only a little less than our total oil imports, and more than twice the energy supplied by all our nuclear power plants.

Materials: processing and packaging of animal foods uses large amounts of strategically important and critically scarce raw materials including aluminum, copper, iron and steel, tin, zinc, potassium, rubber, wood, and petroleum products.

Food resources: 90 percent of our grains and legumes and approximately one half of the fish catch is fed to livestock, while 800 million people are going hungry.

Cost of living: meats generally cost five to six times as much as foods containing an equivalent amount of vegetable protein, and consumption of animal foods adds approximately $4,000 to an average household's annual budget, including the cost of increased medical care.

Employment: production and processing of animal food has led to the centralization and automation of this industry, idling thousands of farm and food workers and small farmers.

International trade: the value of imports of meat and other animal foods, farm machinery fertilizers, and petroleum for production of animal foods is approximately equivalent to our national trade deficit of $40 billion.

Source: Alex Hershaft, Ph.D., "Introductory Statement," A Symposium on the National Impacts of Recommended Dietary Changes (Toronto: American Association for the Advancement of Science, January 4, 1981).

170. Organic vs. Chemical Farming

Nutrients in Organic and Chemically Grown Foods											
	Ash*	P	Ca	Mg	K	Na	Bo	Mn	Fe	Cu	Co
Snap Beans											
Organic	10.45	0.36	40.5	60.0	99.7	8.6	73	60	227	69.0	0.26
Chemical	4.04	0.22	15.5	14.8	29.1	0.0	10	2	10	3.0	0.00
Cabbage											
Organic	10.38	0.38	60.0	43.6	148.3	20.4	42	13	94	48.0	0.15
Chemical	6.12	0.18	17.5	13.6	33.7	0.8	7	2	20	0.4	0.00
Lettuce											
Organic	24.48	0.43	71.0	49.3	176.5	12.2	37	169	516	60.0	0.19
Chemical	7.01	0.22	16.0	13.1	53.7	0.0	6	1	9	3.0	0.00
Tomatoes											
Organic	14.2	0.35	23.0	59.2	148.3	6.5	36	68	1938	53.0	0.63
Chemical	6.07	0.16	4.5	4.5	58.8	0.0	3	1	1	0.0	0.00
Spinach											
Organic	28.56	0.52	96.0	203.9	237.0	69.5	88	117	1584	32.0	0.25
Chemical	12.38	0.27	47.5	46.9	84.6	0.8	12	1	19	0.3	0.20

*Total ash or mineral matter (% of dry weight). Ca through Na show mill equivalents per 100 grams dry weight. Bo through Co show trace elements parts per million dry weight.

Source: Firman E. Baer Report, Rutgers University, 1984.

• Researchers at Rutgers University reported that non-organic produce had as little as 25 percent as much mineral content as organic produce. The scientists compared beans, cabbage, lettuce, tomatoes, and spinach purchased at a supermarket and an organic natural foods store and found substantially higher levels of phosphorous, calcium, magnesium, potassium, sodium, boron, manganese, iron, copper, and cobalt and other minerals and trace elements in the organically grown vegetables.

Source: *Firman E. Baer Report* (New Brunswick, N.J.: Rutgers University, 1984).

Comparison of Organic and Conventional Farming *		
	Organic Farm	Conventional Farm
Surface soil color	Dark grey brown	Grey brown
Polysacchride content (g kg-1)	1.13	1.00
Moisture content (%)	15.49	8.98
Modulus of rupture	1.61 x 10 -2	1.98 x 10 -2
Surface texture	Silt loam	Silk loam
Bulk density (mg m -3)	Silty clay loam	Silty clay loam
Topsoil thickness (cm)	39.80	36.68
Subsoil thickness (cm)	55.60	39.80
Average winter wheat yields (tons ha)	4.50**	4.90
*On adjacent farms in Washington State		
** Researchers noted this was 13% more than another adjacent conventional farm		
Source: Nature, 1987		

• Comparing two neighboring farms in the Palouse region of Washington state, researchers found that the organic farm's topsoil was six inches thicker than the farm using chemical methods. The organic soil also had a softer crust and held more moisture. The scientists concluded that intensive tillage practices associated with continuous monoculture or short rotations of crops may make soils more susceptible to erosion. "This study indicates that, in the long term, the organic farming system was more effective than the conventional farming system in reducing soil erosion and, therefore, in maintaining soil productivity," the investigators concluded.

Source: J. P. Reganold, L. F.Elliott, and Y. L. Unger, "Long-Term Effects of Organic and Conventional Farming on Soil Erosion," *Nature* 330:370-72, 1987.

• A more organic approach to agriculture would not reduce yields or appreciably raise food prices, according to Cornell University researchers. David Pimentel, an entomologist and ecologist at the New York State College of Agriculture and Life Sciences at Cornell, and colleagues analyzed 300 scientific studies and reported that pesticides could be reduced by up to 90 percent without affecting crop yields or the costs of foods. Since the 1940s, pesticide use has multiplied thirty-three times and potency has increased ten times, yet more crops are lost to insects today than fifty years ago. For example, 3.5 percent of the national corn crop was lost to pests then. Today despite a thousand-fold increase in insecticide use, losses have increased to 12 percent. The report also cited other drawbacks to chemicals including the poisoning of 45,000 farm workers and an estimated 6,000 cases of pesticide-induced cancers each year.

Source: David Pimental, *Handbook of Pest Management in Agriculture* (Boca Raton, Fl.: CRC Press, 1991) and Jane Brody, "Using Fewer Pesticides Is Seen as Beneficial," *New York Times*, April 2, 1991.

171. *Alternative Agriculture*

In a landmark report *Alternative Agriculture*, the National Acadmey of Sciences found that "alternative farming methods are practical and economical ways to maintain yields, conserve soil, maintain water quality, and lower operating costs through improved farm management and reduced use of fertilizers and pesticides."

In the 1989 report, the seventeen-member expert panel found that adoption of organic, renewable, sustainable, low-input, and other alternative practices including rotations with legumes and nonleguminous crops, the continued use of improved cultivars, integrated pest management and biological pest control, reduced use of antibiotics in livestock, and lower-cost management strategies that use fewer synthetic chemicals could have substantial "economic benefits to farmers and environmental gains for the nation."

The adverse effects of conventional farming cited include:

• Environmental and occupational health problems resulting from extensive use of synthetic chemical fertilizer and pesticides; agricultural chemicals have been associated with causing cancer, behavioral effects, altered immune system function, and allergic reations.

• Insecticides accounting for 30 percent, herbicides accounting for 50 percent, and fungicides accounting for 90 percent of all agricultural use have been found to cause tumors in laboratory animals.

• Insects, weeds, and pathogens continue to develop resistance to some commonly used insecticides, herbicides, and fungicides.

• Insects and pathogens also continue to overcome inbred genetic resistance of plants; in 1986 more than 440 insect and mite species and more than 70 fungus species were resistant to some pesticides.

• Widespread pesticide use has severely stressed fish, fowl, domestic animals, and wildlife including honeybee and wild bee populations that are vital to the production of vegetables and other crops.

• Chemical agriculture is the leading cause of pollution in surface water and groundwater in many states, affecting an estimated 46 percent of all counties in the U.S.

• The decreasing genetic diversity of many major U.S. crops and livestock species increases potential for sudden widespread losses from disease.

The report was particularly critical of federal grading standards which "discourage alternative pest control practices for fruits and vegetables by imposing cosmetic and insect-part criteria that have little if any relation to nutritional quality. Meat and dairy grading standards continue to provide economic incentives for high-fat content, even though considerable evidence supports the relationship between high consumption of fats and chronic diseases, particularly heart disease."

The report cited the benefits of alternative farming including:

• Increased "environmental and health effects without necessarily decreasing — and in some cases increasing — per acre crop yields."

• Rotating crops often results in yields 10 to 20 percent greater than growing just a single crop regardless of the amount of fertilizer used.

• Organic methods hold water better, improve soil tilth, have a high exchange capacity for binding and relasing some mineral nutrients; serve as a food source for soil microbiotic that recycle soil nutrients, and contribute to remineralization.

Among the case histories presented in the report are the Lundberg Brothers farm in Richvale, California, which grows organic brown rice; the Spray Brothers Farm near Mount Vernon, Ohio, whose crops include organic soybeans and adzuki beans; and the Ferrari Farm near Linden, California, which grows organic vegetables, nuts, and fruits using a natural insect control method based on the sea vegetable kelp.

Source: National Academy of Sciences, *Alternative Agriculture* (Washington, D.C.: National Academy Press, 1989).

172. Diet and Global Warming

• Beef-rich diets contribute to global warming, according to a Dutch study investigating the greenhouse effect. The scientists estimated that 5 percent of the heating up is due to meat and dairy production, especially the spread of cattle pasture and feedlots into carbon-dioxide absorbing forests. Beef intake is six times higher in industrial nations than in nonindustrial nations and is growing 1 percent annually.

Plant sources of protein were recommended as an alternative, and a shift to pork was recommended as a transitional measure. Pork takes from 10 to 30 percent as much feed per protein calorie to produce as beef and produces less methane. Raising chickens was found to add as much to warming as beef and was not advised.

Source: *Science News*, December 9, 1989.

• "Switching from a steak to a vegetable burger" may be one of the most effective way to reduce the Greenhouse Effect, according to a study by the International Project for Sustainable Energy Paths.

"Eating less beef has a double advantage for the climate," reported Florentin Krause, a researcher with the organization which analyzes public policy on energy and the environment. Livestock production takes forest land that contributes to reducing carbon dioxide in the atmosphere and also causes people in Third World countries to use marginal land for producing food.

Livestock production also produces methane, a greenhouse gas that is twenty to thirty times more harmful to the environment than carbon dioxide. According to Krause, cows release about 5 to 9 percent of their food as methane, and animal food production is the single greatest human source of this gas. Altogether, he calculated that beef consumption accounts for 5 to 10 percent of the Greenhouse Effect.

Krause and his co-workers proposed a "climate tax" on beef to encourage people to avoid it and promote a whole foods diet.

Source: F. Krause et al. "Energy Policy in the Greenhouse," Volume One, in *Vegetarian Times*, April 1990.

173. Diet and the Environment

The modern meat-based diet has contributed to environmental destruction. In a survey of leading organizations and individuals in the fields of nutrition and ecology including Frances Moore Lappé, author of *Diet for a Small Planet*; John Robbins, author of *Diet for a New America*; David Pimentel of Cornell University's College of Agriculture; and Robin Hur, an Oregon-based researcher, *Vegetarian Times* summarized findings showing that a whole foods diet could contribute to a healthier planet:

• More than 50 percent of tropical rainforest deforestation (216,000 acres total per day) is linked with livestock production.

• An average of 55 square feet (a small kitchen) of forest is lost for every hamburger produced from cattle raised in former Central American rainforests.

• The current rate of species' extinction from loss of tropical rainforests and related habitats is 1,000 per year.

• One acre of trees is saved each year by each person who switches to a vegan diet.

• The average amount of water required daily for a vegetarian who eats dairy food and eggs is about 1,200 gallons, about 25 percent the amount for someone eating the standard American diet. The amount of water required for a person on a dairy-free vegetarian diet is 300 gallons.

• About 85 percent of the topsoil loss in the U.S. is directly connected with livestock production.

• A reduction in meat consumption by only 10 percent would free enough grain in the U.S. to feed an estimated 60 million people worldwide.

• More than 50 percent of the water pollution in the U.S. is associated with animal food production and chemical farming.

• Imported oil could be cut by 60 percent if the nation switched to a vegetarian diet.

Source: "Is a Burger Worth It?," *Vegetarian Times*, April, 1990, pp. 20-21

174. Rainforest Diet

New discoveries in the Amazon show that the traditional people in the rainforests utilized a sophisticated blend of agriculture and forestry to yield rich harvests and at the same time preserve the delicate ecosystem. The Kayapo of Brazil cultivated circular fields by felling several large trees so that their crowns fell on the periphery of the circle and by planting crops in between. Later the dead trees are burned, the rains wash the ash into the soil, and crops, including corn and rice, are planted in concentric circles.

Source: William K. Stevens, "Research in 'Virgin' Amazon Uncovers Complex Farming,"*New York Times*, Science Section, April 3, 1990.

175. Biological Transmutation

• In 1959 French scientist Louis Kervran started publishing his discoveries in the field of biological transmutation — the synthesis of necessary but unavailable chemical elements out of simpler, available ones. His interest in this field began when he studied workers in the Sahara desert, who excreted more sodium than they consumed. Food tests showed that a comparable excess amount of potassium was being taken. Kervran showed that potassium was capable of being transmuted into sodium in the body.

Developing the theories of George Ohsawa that elements can be transmuted into one another peacefully without smashing the atom, Kervran went on to find that iron could be made from manganese, silica from calcium, and phosphorus from sulfur. Kervran's experiments have wide industrial, scientific, and social applications. For example, biological transmutations could be applied to rendering harmless nuclear wastes, toxic spills, and other chronic environmental hazards.

Source: Louis C. Kervran, *Biological Transmutations* (Brooklyn: Swan House, 1972).

• In 1978 scientists for the U.S. military tested Ohsawa and Kervran's theories of biological transmutation and verified some of their experiments. The researchers concluded that living biological systems are "mini-cyclotrons" that can change one element into another and have a wide range of potential applications in the field of energy production.

Source: S. Goldfein, "Energy Development from Elemental Transmutations in Biological Systems," Report 2247 (Ft. Belvoir, Va.: U.S. Army Mobility Equipment Research and Development Command, 1978).

13

A Healthy,
Peaceful World

In China, the word for peace, wa, combines ideographs for "grain" and "mouth." In India, the Vedic word for war means "desire for cows." Ancient people in the East intuitively knew that eating whole grains made for a healthy, peaceful society, while eating excessive animal food made for personal and social disorder. In the West, the legend of Lost Paradise attributed a happy, peaceful past to a simple grain-and-vegetable way of life. According to Ovid, the Roman poet: "Golden was that first age which, with no one to compel, without a law, of its own will, kept faith and did the right. . . . There was no need at all of armed men, for nations, secure from war's alarms, passed the years in gentle ease. The earth herself, without compulsion, untouched by hoe or plowshare, of herself gave all things needful. And men, content with food which came with no one's seeking, gathered . . . [Nature's] stores of grain, and the fields, though unfallowed, grew white with the heavy bearded wheat." In Plato's The Republic, *Socrates argues that a plant-quality diet is essential to keeping the peace. Modern anthropological, sociological, and historical studies are confirming the wisdom of the past.*

176. Peace in Traditional Societies

• A study of megalithic culture, including cave drawings and stone tools, shows no evidence of weapons of war or organized social aggression by one group against another. War also seems to be unknown in the earliest civilization. "[I]t would seem that peaceful behavior is really typical of mankind when living simple lives such as those of the food-gatherers. If that be accepted, it follows that man must somehow or other have become warlike as human culture developed. . . Not only does the Old Stone Age fail to reveal any definite signs of weapons, but the earliest of the predynastic Egyptians also evidently were peaceful. They made maces, which may or may not have been weapons, but very few of them have been found in their graves. Similarly, the first settlements at Susa and Anau have yielded evidence that the people were peaceful."

Source: W. J. Perry, *The Growth of Civilization*, pp. 194-96.

• In northeastern Thailand, archaeologists have recently found evidence of a bronze-age culture much older than that of the Tigris and Euphrates Valley in ancient Mesopotamia, which has been believed until recently to be the cradle of civilization. By 3600 B.C., the Ban Chiang people, as they are known, lived in permanent villages, grew rice, wove silk for clothing, and wore bronze jewelry. According to scientists, they must have learned bronze-making much earlier because the ratio of copper to tin in their work is in the exact proportion of maximum durability that took metalworkers three thousand years to perfect in the Middle East. Unlike later civilizations in Mesopotamia, they appear to have been entirely peaceful and did not use their advanced technology for destructive purposes. Analysis of more than one hundred skeletons unearthed found no deaths by violence, and no weapons of war have been discovered.

Source: Ronald Schiller, "Where Was the 'Cradle of Civilization?'" *Reader's Digest*, August 1980, pp. 67-71.

• In the American Midwest, recent excavations at Koster, seventy miles north of St. Louis, have revealed the outlines of a prehistoric Native American culture that occupied the site peacefully for 9,500 years. The inhabitants of Koster lived on wild cereal-like seeds, water lotus, hickory nuts, deer, fish, and other wild plants and animals. They had tools for grain and vegetable processing, as well as baskets and leatherwork. By 5000 B.C., they were living in permanent wooden houses and establishing long-term villages. Until about A.D. 800, when they came into contact with highly complex Mississippian cultures and were overrun, they is no sign of invasion or violent death.

Source: Stuart Struever and Felicia Holton, *Koster* (New York: Anchor, 1979).

• According to anthropologists, warfare was unknown among many primitive societies including the Andaman Islanders, the Arunta, the Eskimos, the Mission Indians, the Semang, the Todas, the Western Shoshoni, the Yahgan, and the Australian Aborigines.

Source: Alexander Lesser, "War and the State," in Morton Fried, Marvin Harris, and Robert Murphy, editors, *War: The Anthropology of Armed Conflict and Aggression* (Garden City: American Museum of Natural History, 1968), pp. 213-36.

177. War in Primitive Society

Described as the "meanest and most unlikeable people on earth," the majority of the Qolla Indians in rural Peru engage in murder, rape, arson, fighting and stealing and other criminal behavior. In one village of over 1000, researchers found that over 50 percent of household heads were directly or indirectly involved with violent death and murder. Dr. Ralph Bolton tested the blood sugar of all males in the village and found that over 50 percent were clinically hypoglycemic. To keep their blood sugar levels up, the Qolla frequently drank alcohol and chewed coca.

Source: R. Bolton, *Aggression in Qolla Society* (Champaign: Garland Press, 1978).

178. Food and Social Violence

In a symposium on the anthropology of armed conflict and aggression, Margaret Mead suggested that social measures necessary for the prevention of modern warfare might include "radical changes in diet." "It might be that the production of a social environment in which there were no living creatures used as food . . . might be sufficient to extinguish the human capacity to kill living things, or, alternatively, might make it socially impossible to modulate and teach the difference between permitted and impermissible killing either of other living things or of other human beings."

Source: Margaret Mead, "Alternatives to War," in Morton Fried, Marvin Harris, and Robert Murphy, editors, *War: The Anthropology of Armed Conflict and Aggression* (Garden City: American Museum of Natural History, 1968), pp. 213-36.

179. Diet and the Napoleonic Wars

"Napoleon's armies took white bread with them wherever they

went in Europe as a banner of liberation from old dull bran or rye breads."

Source: Hugh Thomas, *A History of the World* (New York: Harper & Row, 1979), p. 386.

Wars of Modern Civilization by 50-Year Periods 1480-1941									
State	1480-1550	1550-1600	1600-1650	1650-1700	1700-1750	1750-1800	1800-1850	1850-1900	1900-1941	Total
England	6	6	7	10	8	7	14	13	7	78
France	10	10	6	8	4	4	11	12	6	71
Spain	12	7	11	6	7	5	6	7	3	64
Russia	2	6	7	8	7	10	10	4	7	61
Austria	13	4	3	8	7	5	6	3	3	52
Turkey	6	5	5	4	3	5	5	5	5	43
Poland	3	4	7	5	3	2	1	1	4	30
Sweden	2	6	4	4	5	3	2	0	0	26
Italy	0	0	4	1	5	2	1	5	7	25
Germany	0	1	1	3	4	4	2	3	5	23
Netherlands	1	1	2	8	5	2	2	0	2	23
Denmark	2	1	3	5	1	3	3	1	1	20
United States	0	0	0	0	0	2	4	2	5	13
China	0	0	0	1	0	0	0	4	6	11
Japan	0	0	0	0	0	0	0	2	7	9
World	32	31	34	30	18	20	41	48	24	278

Source: A Study of War, 1965

180. Diet and War

In *A Study of War,* the century's major survey of the origin and cause of conflict, Quincy Wright, an authority in the field of international law and adviser to the U.S. War Department and the Nuremberg Tribunal, concluded that war — especially civilized war in which the taking of human life is a primary objective — is unnatural and that "the trend of evolution has been toward symbiotic relations and perhaps toward vegetarian diet."

After researching the incidence of human aggression in nearly six hundred primitive cultures, Professor Wright concluded that warfare is more prevalent among societies in which animal food forms a major part of the diet than in societies in which a more vegetarian way of life is practiced. He further arranged the twenty-six historical civilizations from ancient to modern times according to degrees of warlikeness, based on twenty-five variables including general social characteristics, frequency of battles, military techniques, and military characteristics. Once again, according to his listing, the vegetarian and semi-vegetarian civilizations generally fall into the peaceful category, while those in which substantial amounts of meat, poultry, fish, or other animal food was consumed tended to be warlike.

He also ranked modern civilizations according to the number of wars fought in the last five centuries and found that the Western meat-eating countries, led by England, were involved in the most wars, while cereal and plant-based countries, such as China and Japan, went to war least often.

Source: Quincy Wright, *A Study of War*, second edition (Chicago: University of Chicago Press, 1965).

181. Diet and Peace in Lebanon

In 1975 Susana Sarué left the Sorbonne in Paris where she was completing her doctorate in nutrition to travel to the Middle East to care for Rema Cheblis, a young Lebanese girl with a fatal brain tumor. The girl's condition improved on a macrobiotic diet, but one day she glimpsed herself in a mirror and saw for the first time that she had no hair and that one eye socket was empty where the tumor pressed against it. She lost the will to live, stopped eating, and passed away peacefully.

Rema's parents asked Susana to stay and help restore peace between waring Christians and Moslems in Beirut, as well as Palestinian refugees caught in the fighting, and Israeli soldiers and officials. Susana investigated and found that there used to be a whole grain bread in Lebanon called Wise Bread because it gave wisdom, or nourishment, but for many years the bread had been made entirely with white flour. This flat bread composed about two-thirds of the daily diet. With donations, they opened a small bakery and brought the bread to the homes of families who had a lot of children and who didn't have any work. Gradually people learned how to make the bread themselves. Later, a natural foods cooperative was set up and made grains, beans, miso, tamari soy sauce, and other healthy foods available. Stephen Malkonian, an agronomist who worked with a pesticide company, became involved after relieving migraine headaches he had suffered from for years in only ten days. He set up an organic agricultural project on 25 hectares of land near the Syrian border and planted grains, vegetables, fruits, and nuts.

In Beirut, some Catholic priests who heard about the distribution of bread set up a macrobiotic center called Our Home. In East Beirut, Mary Naccour, a prominent journalist who had a two-hour radio program broadcast throughout the Arab world, began to work in the villages and eventually became the leading macrobiotic teacher after Susana returned home. "Other countries — America, France — send us donations: canned food, sugar, white flour, margarine," Naccour observed. "And they send us free medication. It's a vicious circle — the food is eaten, the people get sick, they go to hospitals, they take the medications. The food is eaten, the people beocme more aggressive, angry, and warlike. And the people who send this junk food and medication, the synthetic clothing, also send the bombs. It is also they who say they want to make peace. But the war itself wants to fight because there is war in our hearts and minds."

Source: Michio Kushi and Alex Jack, *One Peaceful World* (New York: St. Martin's Press, 1987), pp. 249-55.

182. Diet and Unity in a Columbian Village

In Virareka, a small village in Colombia, a sugarcane plantation had displaced local farms and fields. Over the years, large amounts of chemicals were applied to the cane, which came to displace all other crops. Deserts replaced green fields of grains and vegetables. Almost all the food eaten locally was brought in and consisted mainly of white flour, sugar, dairy food, meat, and other highly processed foods.

Nutritionist Suana Sarué, a native of Latin America, returned to Colombia to do field work in the 1970s and investigated malnutrition in Virareka. Observing the local chickens which were the most healthy and energetic inhabitants of the village, she noticed they were eating soy grits and sorghum. This insight led her to devise a whole range of foods made from natural ingedients but which looked and tasted like the prestige foods the upper classes ate.

She introduced a variety of cutlets, burgers, and other "meats" with a soya base, offered the people soy milk instead of dairy, and made an ice cream from sorghum and soya. The children's condition began to improve quickly. They became more alert and intelligent in school and less famished. They no longer had large stomachs. They also became more active. A health food bar was opened and managed by the local people. One day, the men of the village went on strike, and the bosses at the sugar plantation refused their demands, reasoning that they would starve after the third day and return to work. But the strikers, subsisting on local grains and beans and soy products, continued for two weeks, and the company was forced to give in and raise their wages.

Source: Michio Kushi and Alex Jack, *One Peaceful World* (New York: St. Martin's Press, 1987), pp. 255-57.

183. A Healthy, Reunified Germany

In 1979, Hildegard Lilienthal, a German nurse, entered a hospital in a suburb of Frankfurt. For years she had been suffering from crippling rheumatism, arthritis, and a heart condition and could no longer walk, work, or care for her family. When medical treatment offered no relief. After several months of eating brown rice, miso soup, and other macrobiotic foods, and applying a hot ginger compress on her kidneys, intestines, and arms and legs, she could walk again and was no longer confined to her home.

Her sons, Uli and Jorj, soon began following her way of eating, but her husband, Hans, continued to like sausage, eggs, cheese, and typical German foods. However, he had poor circulation in his leg, and doctors told him that he would require amputation below the thigh. Hildegard and her sons brought brown rice and other foods to him in the hospital and gave him ginger compresses. Circulation was restored, and he did not need the operation. The manager of a large mining company, Hans later quit his job and joined the rest of the family in teaching macrobiotics and setting up Atlantis, a small tofu and tempeh factory in the family's home.

"By improving people's health, their mentality will change and peace will come to a divided Germany. That is our dream," Hans observed in 1985. Since then, thousands of Germans, Austrians, Swiss, and other Europeans have studied and been helped by the

Lilienthal family, and the Habichtswald Clinic, a cancer clinic in Kassel, a city two hours north of Frankfurt, has begun offering macrobiotic food and home remedies to its patients.

Source: Michio Kushi and Alex Jack, *One Peaceful World* (New York: St. Martin's Press, 1987), pp. 273-78.

184. Diet and Ecology in the Soviet Union

In 1985, Lidia Yamchuk and Hanif Shaimardanov, medical doctors in Cheljabinsk, organized Longevity, the first macrobiotic association in the Soviet Union. At their hospital, they have used dietary methods and acupuncture to treat many patients, especially those suffering from leukemia, lymphoma, and other disorders associated with exposure to nuclear radiation. Since the early 1950s, wastes from Soviet weapons production were dumped into Karachay Lake in Cheljabinsk, an industrial city about 900 miles east of Moscow.

In Leningrad, Yuri Stavitsky, a young pathologist and medical instructor, volunteered as a radiologist in Chernobyl after the nucelar accident on April 26, 1986. Since then, like many disaster workers, he suffered symptoms associated with radiation disease, including tumors of the thyroid. "Since beginning macrobiotics," he reported, "my condition has greatly improved."

In Leningrad, in 1990, a visiting delegation of macrobiotic teachers from the United States, Japan, Germany, and Yugoslavia gave macrobiotic lectures at the Cardiology Center, the Institute of Cytology (the main cancer research center), and the State Institute for the Continuing Education of Doctors. Zoya Tchoueva, a Leningrad psychiatrist and medical researcher, is translating Michio Kushi's book, *The Cancer-Prevention Diet*, into Russian.

In Pushkin, the former country estate of the Russian emperors and a children's convalescent center, town officials and the Agricultural Institute of Leningrad, invited the macrobiotic association to set up an Ecological Village and donated 100 acres of land for organic production of grains and vegetables. Soviet medical and environmental groups such as Union Chernobyl and Peace to the Children of the World hope to begin distributing miso, sea vegetables, and other macrobiotic-quality foods that may help protect against the effects of harmful nuclear radiation.

Source: Alex Jack, "Soviets Embrace Macrobiotics," *One Peaceful World*, Autumn/Winter, 1990.

185. Return to Paradise

For over forty years, Masanobu Fukuoka has devoted himself to natural farming. His methods of raising crops without cultivation, chemicals, and even organic compost have resulted in high yields, fertile strains of seed, and improved quality of the soil.

"In my experience, after the seeds are scattered, crops will grow without cultivation, weeding, fertilizer, or pruning," he explained. "Because different kinds of plants are mixed together, they do not attract the birds, insects, or other pests that commonly invade gardens and farms cultivated with only one variety. Tractors and other heavy machinery that compact and harden the soil are a major cause of erosion and infertility. They destroy microorganisms and other small life that build up the tilth of the soil."

Since publication of his book *The One-Straw Revolution*, he has increasingly devoted himself to global problems. On a visit to Somalia, Ethiopia, and other drought-striken areas of Africa, he discovered that people traditionally used natural farming methods.

In experiments in his native Japan, Fukuoka devised a method to revegetate barren lands by sowing seeds in clay pellets. The pellets are prepared by mixing the seeds of green manure trees, such as acacia that grow in areas of minimal rainfall, and the seeds of clover and alfalfa with grain and vegetable seeds. The mixture of seeds is coated first with a layer of soil, then one of clay, to form clay pellets containing microbes. These completed pellets can then be scattered over the deserts and savannahs. Once scattered, the seeds will not sprout until rain has fallen and conditions for germination are right. Nor will they be eaten by insects, birds, or mice.

"To restore green belts in Africa, seed mixtures can be scattered from airplanes," he proposed. "If this method proves successful, I would like to see the air forces of the world distribute seeds across desertified regions of the planet on a vast scale. Let's launch seeds from the air, not missiles. Freedom and peace with the land begin with natural farming methods. Grains and trees know no artificial boundaries. . . . Everthing starts from the family garden. Through natural farming, the destructive course of civilization can be changed. Once again, the earth can be transformed into a paradise of peace and happiness with enough food for everyone."

Source: Mananobu Fukuoka, "Bringing Back the Rains," *Return to Paradise*, Winter 1988-89, p. 16.

Appendix

Standard Macrobiotic Dietary Guidelines*

Foods for Daily Consumption

• **Whole Cereal Grains:** The principal food of each meal is ideally whole cereal grain, comprising from 50 to 60 percent of the total volume. Whole grains include brown rice, whole wheat berries, barley, millet, and rye, as well as corn, buckwheat, and other botanically similar plants. From time to time, whole grain products, such as cracked wheat, rolled oats, noodles, pasta, bread, baked goods, and other unrefined flour products, may be served as part of this volume.

• **Soup:** One to two small bowls of soup, making up about 5 to 10 percent of daily food intake, are consumed each day. The soup broth is made frequently with miso or tamari soy sauce and also includes vegetable, bean, and grain soups.

• **Vegetables:** About 25 to 30 percent of daily food includes fresh vegetables prepared in a variety of ways, including steaming, boiling, baking, sautéing, salads, and marinades. The vegetables include a variety of root vegetables (such as cabbage, carrots, and daikon radish), ground vegetables (such as onions and fall- and winter-season squashes), and leafy green vegetables (such as kale, collard greens, broccoli, turnip greens, mustard greens, and watercress).

• **Beans and Sea Vegetables:** A small portion, about 10 percent by volume, of daily food intake includes cooked beans such as adzukis, lentils, and chickpeas or bean products such as tofu, tempeh, and natto and sea vegetables, including kombu, wakame, nori, dulse, hijiki, and arame.

• **Seasoning and Oil:** Naturally processed sea salt is used in seasoning, along with miso, tamari soy sauce, umeboshi, brown rice vinegar, fresh grated ginger and other traditional items. Naturally processed, unrefined vegetable oil is recommended for daily cooking such as dark sesame seed oil. Kuzu is commonly used for gravies and sauces.

• **Condiments:** Condiments include gomashio (roasted sesame salt), roasted seaweed powders, umeboshi plums, tekka root vegetable, and many others.

• **Pickles:** A small volume of home-made pickles is eaten each day to aid in digestion of grains and vegetables.

• **Beverages:** Spring or well water is used for drinking, preparing tea, and for general cooking. Bancha twig tea (also known as kukicha) is the most commonly served beverage, though roasted barley tea, and other grain-based teas or traditional, nonstimulant herbal teas are also used frequently.

Occasional Foods for Those in Usual Good Health

• **Animal Food:** A small volume of white-meat fish or seafood may be eaten a few times per week.

• **Seeds and Nuts:** Seeds and nuts, lightly roasted and salted with sea salt or seasoned with tamari soy sauce, may be enjoyed as occasional snacks.

• **Fruit:** Fruit may be taken a few times a week, preferably cooked or naturally dried, as a snack or dessert, provided the fruit grows in the local or similar climate zone.

• **Dessert:** Occasional desserts may consist of cookies, pudding, cake, pie, and other dishes made with naturally sweet foods such as apples, fall and winter squashes, azuki beans, or dried fruit or may be sweetened with a natural grain-based sweetener such as rice syrup, barley malt, or amasake.

---

* These guidelines are for four-season temperate climates of the world including most of the United States, Europe, the U.S.S.R., and China. Recommendations will vary for colder, polar or semi-polar regions and for warmer, tropical or subtropical climates and environments. Way of eating suggestions also include preparing food in an attractive manner, eating with a calm, peaceful mind, and thorough chewing.

Glossary

Atherosclerosis A form of arteriosclerosis in which hardened plaque from fat and cholesterol builds up on the inner walls of arteries, narrowing them and reducing the flow of blood; the underlying cause of most heart attacks and strokes.

Beta-carotene A precursor to Vitamin A that is associated with reduced risk of cancer, heart disease, and other sicknesses. Foods naturally high in beta-carotene are the orange and yellow vegetables such as carrots, squash, dark green vegetables such as kale, broccoli, and Chinese cabbage, and orange fruits such as apricots, peaches, and cantaloupe.

Cholesterol A waxy constituent of all animal fats and oils, which can contribute to heart disease, cancer, and other illnesses. Vegetable-quality foods do not contain cholesterol. The liver naturally produces all the serum cholesterol needed by the body.

Complex carbohydrates Starches or sugars in whole grains, vegetables, seaweeds, and fruits that are gradually metabolized and supply a slow, steady source of energy and nutrients.

Cruciferous vegetables Dark green leafy vegetables that are associated with reduced risk of cancer including broccoli, cabbage, Brussels sprouts, kohlrabi, kale, cauliflower, mustard greens, rutabaga, and turnips.

Fiber The part of whole grains, vegetables, and fruits that is not broken down in digestion and gives bulk to wastes.

Lactovegetarian A vegetarian who eats dairy products. An ovolactovegetarian eats both eggs and dairy products. A vegan avoids all animal foods and products.

Miso A fermented paste made from soybeans, sea salt, and usually barley or rice. Used in soups, stews, spreads, and as a seasoning, miso gives a nice sweet taste and salty flavor.

Natural foods Whole foods that are unrefined and untreated with artificial additives or preservatives.

Organic foods Food grown without the use of chemical fertilizers, herbicides, pesticides, or other artificial sprays.

Polyunsaturated fats Essential fatty acids found in high concentrations in whole grains, beans, seeds, and a lesser extent in fish.

Saturated fats Fats found primarily in meats, poultry, eggs, dairy food, and a few vegetable oils such as coconut and palm tree oil, which raise serum cholesterol and contribute to atherosclerosis.

Sea vegetables An edible seaweed such a kombu, wakame, arame, hiziki, nori, or dulse.

Tempeh A soy product made from split soybeans, water, and a special bacteria; high in protein with a rich, dynamic taste, tempeh is used in soups, stews, sandwiches, casseroles, and other dishes.

Tofu Soybean curd made from soybeans and nigari; high in protein and prepared in cakes and used in soups, vegetable dishes, salads, sauces, dressings, and other dishes.

Umeboshi A salted pickled plum that has aged usually for several years; used as a seasoning, a condiment, and as a medicine.

Whole grains Unrefined cereal grains to which nothing has been added or subtraced in milling except for the inedible outer hull. Whole grains include brown rice, millet, barley, whole wheat, oats, rye, buckwheat, and corn.

Index

and migraines, 79-80
nutritional status of, 22, 32-33,
123, 127
in prison, 129
and radiation, 87-89
and sports, 110-11
magnesium, 36, 73, 133
Maimonides, Moses, 15
malaria, 115
malnutrition, 98-99
McCarrison, Robert, 18
McGovern, George, 25, 116
Mead, Margaret, 142
measles, 77
meat
and cancer, 55, 59-60, 86
consumption of, 24
guidelines for use of, 25-40
harmful effects, 17, 23, 69, 81, 86,
108, 110, 124
substitutes for, 37-38
useable protein of, 131
meditation, 42, 49
melanoma, 65, 66
menstruation, 38
mental illness, 116-19
Mexico, 23
Middle East, 15, 141, 144-45
migraine, 79-80, 99, 145
milk, 19, 24, 36, 47, 85
and allergies, 67, 68
and calcium, 82, 83
and cancer, 53, 55, 56
and children, 124
and iron, 77
and juvenile delinquency, 127-28
and protein quality, 107-08, 131
millet, 12, 60, 77, 125, 149
miso
and B$_{12}$, 106, 107
and cancer, 57, 64, 86, 92
and cerebrovascular disease, 64
guidelines for use of, 149, 150
and heart disease, 51, 64, 86
and high blood pressure, 64, 86
in a hospital, 125

and intestinal disorders, 76
medicinal use of, 16, 146
nutritional value of, 78, 82
and radiation, 86, 89, 91-92, 147
and sexuality, 112
MIT, 116
Mizuno, Namboku, 17
modern medicine, 9-10
monounsaturated fats, 26, 27, 51
motion sickness, 80
Multiple Risk Factor Intervention
Trial, 51-52
multiple sclerosis, 80-81
mustard greens, 29, 77, 82, 83, 149
Nagasaki, 87-88, 92
Napoleon, 142-43
National Academy of Sciences, 29,
35, 40, 53, 85, 108, 135
National Cancer Institute, 53
Native Americans, 23, 72, 141
natto, 57, 76, 78, 82, 150
natural agriculture, 148
natural immunity, 93-100
navy beans, 46, 59, 82
Netherlands, 47, 105, 137, 143
New England Journal of Medicine, 43,
44, 49, 54, 60, 104, 108
Newbold, Vivien, 66
Ni-Hon-San Study, 45
niacin, 36, 73
nightshades, 84
nori, 56, 77, 82, 150
Norway, 59
nuclear fallout, 87-92, 147
nuclear power, 132
nuclear wastes, 139
Nutrition and Cancer, 57, 58, 64, 115
nuts, 21, 61, 82, 85, 125, 150
oats, 24, 77, 85
obesity, 21, 23, 32, 33, 35, 39, 81
Ohsawa, George, 19-20, 89, 139
oil, 34, 36, 66, 80, 81, 150
Okinawa, 53
onions, 149
organic farming, 131, 133-34
Ornish, Dean, 40, 49-50